TEETH
IN MORTAL
COMBAT

TEETH
IN MORTAL
COMBAT

HOW TO Unleash
Your Basic Instinct
FOR SURVIVAL

LESTER SAWICKI, D.D.S.

Teeth in Mortal Combat
How to Unleash Your Basic Instinct for Survival

5501A Balcones Dr #155, Austin, TX 78731
www.Tooth-Fight.com
www.Revolutiontooth.com
info@revolutiontooth.com

Library of Congress Number: 2010903469
ISBN: 9780984370627

Interior Art by Li Zhang
Cover Design by Perry Taylor
Interior Design by William Groetzinger

Dedicated to my father,
Marian Sawicki

&

In loving memory of my
mother, Irena Sawicki
01–23–1926 to 09–26–1981

CONTENTS

Contents

CONTENTS

PART FOUR... *Lightning and Thunder*

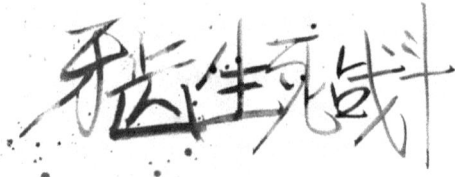

牙达生元战斗

Tooth Fight!

Do Not Conform!
Lest you turn into heartless stone.
Be Radical!
Cut your tooth
on freedom's path.
Tongue as ruthless as an axe.

Through thick fog
in search of truth
fearless minds clash.
Teeth of sensei lunge, snarl, and gnash.

Let no assailant bash
your holy diamond teeth.
Not any aggressor's golden fist,
nor iron feet.

Stink your steel jaw with blood-sudored
dark enemies gnawed into grist.
Snap the backbone, tear out the jugular,
molarized bile crushed into spit.

Spirit driven to survive
Fierce Hoopla! is its chosen style
Teeth in Mortal Combat, be
No Think—Instinct.

...Lester Sawicki, D.D.S.

"During my thirty-three years of dental practice, I have examined and interviewed a number of patients between 85 and 100 years old. I was amazed by their grace, agility, mental acuity, vitality, enthusiasm, and overall health. The healthiest among them had managed to retain most of their teeth through superior oral health care practices. A few could easily crack walnuts. This convinces me... there is a definite connection between good oral health and a healthy long life."

The Teeth Whitening Cure, 2009
www.RevolutionTooth.com

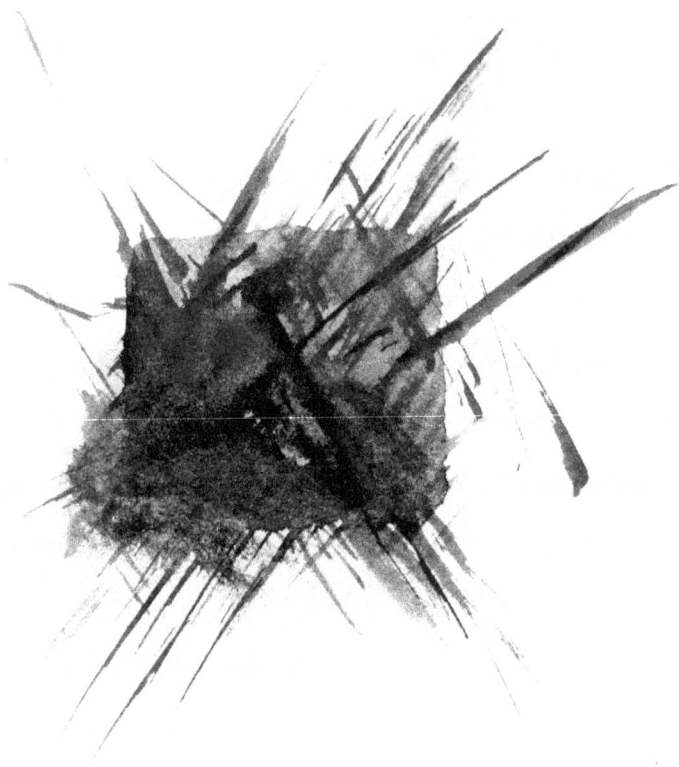

PREFACE

As a seasoned practitioner of martial arts and meditation—and a student of the connection between healthy
teeth and a vibrant long life—I asked myself what bearing teeth had on my martial arts and meditation practice.
A series of small, serendipitous thoughts led to personal
insights which further ignited a powerful epiphany. In many
respects, this epiphany was as shocking as it was enlighten-
ing, and the thought processes involved were somewhat
radical and 'outside of the box.'

Mark my words in this: the conformist shackles his self-
progress. The open-minded rebel cuts a path of discovery
with a sword honed by hard questions. Therefore, I dare not
add to the dust on your mirror. The few words I use will not
place you in harm's way, and the following dissertation will
be brief, painted within a fog of misty clouds. The fiery sun
within you is more than capable of burning through these
humble, perhaps meaningless revelations. The only advice
given is that you FIGHT tooth and nail to Lift the Veil of
Mystery.

Lifting the Veil of Mystery is a ritual practiced by all
would be martial artists. You have chosen this moment in
time to be here with me, to catch a glimpse behind the veil.
I honor you for that, and will share some of my very personal experiences and treasures discovered in the practice
of martial arts: Perfection as a goal can paralyze movement.
The path is a journey of error. Questions chisel away the
multiple coverings of fear; by becoming aware of one's fear,
transformation can happen; fear does not transform into its

opposite, bravery; when you accept your fear, the transformation is respect for your power and the fear slowly disappears. To become a Master—"There is no answer."

In my opinion, the blinding snow laden mountains of martial art styles, as some may claim, do not have a unifying original source. There is no single rooted tree of self-defense from which all the others sprang and branched out. We find no one movement that is simple, pure, undiluted, and therefore, more powerful and effective than all the others. What we do find in the turbulent, snowy, wind-swept mountain peaks is Stillness—from which all forms arise. It has no name.

Think of a wintry blue sky thick with snow clouds that condense and crystallize the first original snowflakes. Which snowflake hits the solid earth first to hold the distinction of being the Authentic One? Is that the 'snowflake' we should try to emulate in our martial arts fighting style? Is that the singular form that holds the superior wisdom, strength, and effectiveness we are searching for? Clouds do not vie for the title of "Creator of First Snowflake," nor do snow flakes fall from the sky competing to be the first to land on earth. It is IMPOSSIBLE to imagine the very first snowflake that gently touched earth's highest mountain peak. Were humans there to discover, preserve, and catalog it? Who today can claim and prove direct lineage to this venerable form? Yet importantly, the snow crystals do, in their floating dance downward to solid ground, travel together. They all grow in synchrony, each having a unique and intricate design with recognizable symmetry.

And likewise with martial arts, I believe we waste precious time arguing one fighting style's superiority over another. There is no single original martial art that is more effective and deadly than those that have followed. There is no one movement that defeats all others. When discussing and comparing various martial art styles, you might as well be talking about snowflakes.

What piques my curiosity is that something appears to exist behind the common symmetry of all martial arts styles. For lack of a better word, I call it "instinct." Humans today still depend on instinct for survival; it is the basis for all self-defense when engaged in Mortal Combat. And in this book I reveal an instinct common to all, from infant to adult. It is this distinct instinct that sparks all the necessary forces needed to recreate human life. Beginning at birth it feeds, protects, and preserves us until the day we decide to pass from this earth... This instinct, along with many more pearls of information, is revealed in this book where you will discover Survival Instincts Hidden Behind the Secret Smile of Laughing Buddha. As an added hidden bonus, you will learn why I believe "Molar Combat with Killer White Teeth and Massive Jaws" may be a Secret to Immortality.

Based on my own experience, I believe society can depress, deform, corrupt, and mutate an individual's elemental expression of instinct. Instinct breathes life into the symmetry that exists in all of us, yet today dwells suppressed, crippled, or dormant in most of us. In this book I try to illuminate and release our birthright to an instinct nearly buried today among society's artificial constructs. I hope that after reading this book you will have a greater understanding of what it means to truly live FREE as a human being—with the freedom to express your most basic instinct for survival.

I sincerely hope that the turbulent joys and sorrows that have arisen from my twenty-five year study of the mysteries of the East will benefit you many times over.

Lester Sawicki, DDS

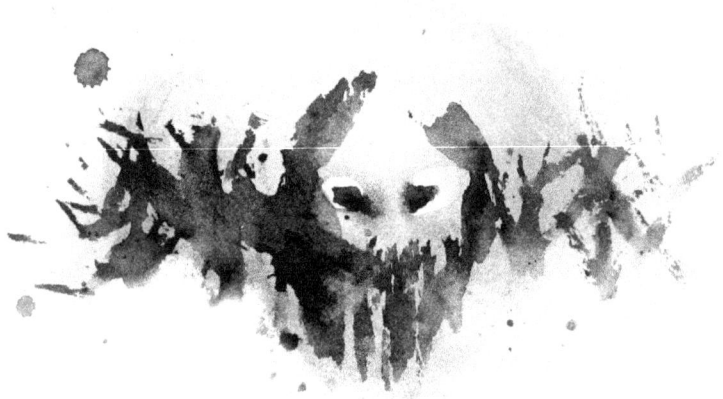

PROLOGUE

If you are one of the hundreds of thousands of aspiring martial artists studying hard under the tutelage of a Master, you have most certainly heard and read the following tenets many times:

A.) The lowest level of victory over an opponent is through the use of muscular strength alone.

B.) The middle level utilizes and releases one's intrinsic energy, or chi, as a kite on a string.

C.) At the highest level one projects the spirit at the opponent and they therefore dare not take any aggressive action.

Some Martial Art Masters in the United States of America have a rule of thumb stating that it takes twenty years of consistent practice in each of the three levels in order to boil the cauldron of ignorance into the steam of wizardry. That means a minimum of sixty years of consistent, methodical, focused, blood, guts, sweat, and tears training is required in the pursuit of Lifting the Veil of Mystery.

In my experience and observation over the last fifty years, few Americans (myself included) have gone beyond a mere warming of the pot in level "A." Many have become sick, disabled, or died during their quest for Mastery of level "B" (sadly, some were friends). I am sure that you will also agree that Level "C" has been reduced for the majority to nothing more than myths exchanged over beer, coffee, and healing teas.

But it is worth noting that some of the Asian Masters who travel to the West to demonstrate and teach martial arts are not bound by this Twenty Year Golden Rule of Time. Many of them—some under the age of thirty-five and a few barely in their late teens—can readily demonstrate all three levels. What is the truth behind mastering the three levels? Where are the answers?

Many mysteries may be solved in states of deep relaxation and heavy dreams. I should not have been surprised then, when it was during such a state that my cauldron began to lightly steam, misting a few fleeting answers to my conscious mind. The veil of mystery began to flutter, if not lift. But I was surprised—AND angry! The scenario was not presenting itself as expected. In fact, the whole scene seemed to be running in reverse. However, my experience gleaned from scars scalded by burning sweat—in concert with these revelations—helped to transmute my anger into the discovery of Hex-Diamond White Teeth & Predator X Jaw and the realization that they are critical to mastering a long life and perhaps even another path to immortality.

I cannot claim that the reading of this book will make your path toward enlightenment any easier or quicker. My prayer is that it brings into your life blossoms of a more fragrant flower!

PART ONE

GATHERING STORM CLOUDS

1

Original Chi

Evolutionists contend that man is descended from prehistoric creatures of sea, sky, and land. The first martial artists were profound philosophers who understood this long ago. The innate energy of each animal was visualized and meditated upon by the first Masters. They devised the Animal Form fighting styles in order to imitate and learn from these creatures, as each animal has specialized instincts for survival that are perfect for that animal's body shape, build, capability, and personality. They learned that studying and practicing Animal Forms could activate latent but powerful animal instincts embedded in man's DNA.

After much dedicated study and practice, an animal's natural power may be tapped to invigorate the practitioner's chi. What was once dormant, due to societal constraints, becomes a vital force behind the martial artist's expression of chi. If one can engage all of the animal energy within oneself, a formidable warrior emerges. One must dive deep into the bubbling well of animal forms to locate the source, but if one pays homage to it, the being quickens and everything seems possible. All dangers dissolve.

Let us review some of the animal forms.
Dragon
Tiger
Snake
Crane

Leopard
Deer
Monkey
Bear
Elephant
Lion
Horse

All of these animals, with the exception of the crane, use their teeth and jaws in combat. And the crane, of course, uses its beak to stab. Elephants use teeth and tusks. The tusks are actually specialized upper incisors, or front teeth, and the elephant has six teeth which are replaced several times throughout its life, a characteristic shared with sharks. Deer have surprisingly powerful bites and, having latched on to their opponent, shake their heads and tear in the manner of pit bulls. The Komodo Dragon, the world's largest lizard, delivers a powerful bite with its serrated teeth and it has been recently discovered that they also utilize a powerful venom to bring down their victims. Monkeys maul with their canines and front teeth. Horses are also tenacious biters.

And it is an undeniable fact that in the early ages of mankind, formidable teeth and jaws were often crucial for survival. Teeth functioned as tools to help create body coverings as animal hides were softened by working the teeth and jaws. Self-defense often depended on the most basic weapon—*sharp teeth and strong jaws*—long before man learned to build weapons. Yet to this day, men, women and children will use their teeth and jaws in mortal combat to best their assailant, be it man or beast.

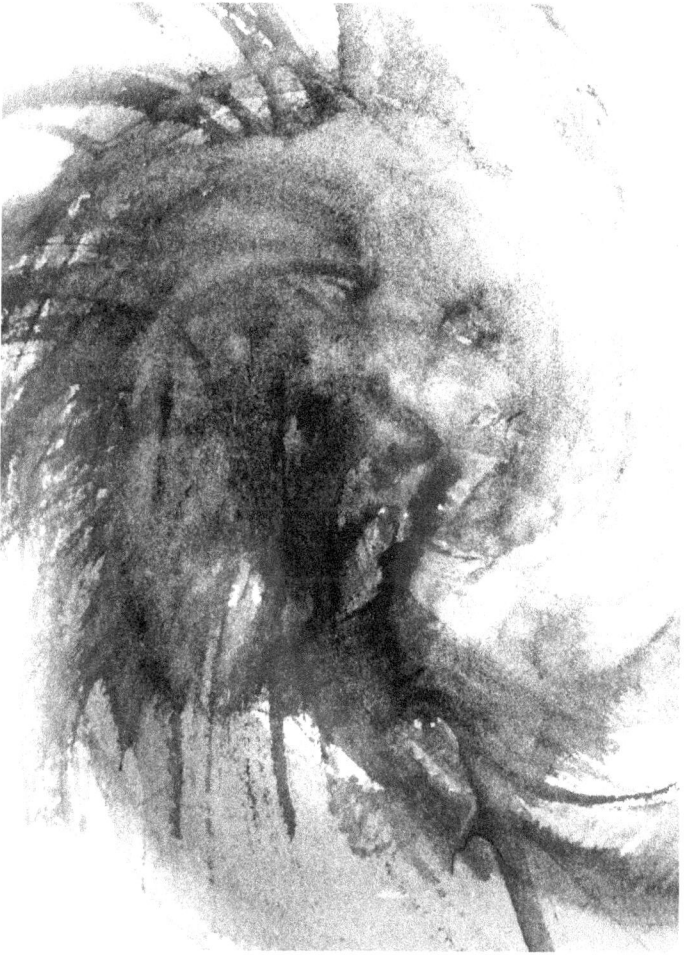

2

Teeth—Our Most Primitive and Primary Weapons of Choice?

1. Teeth are Man's Most Basic Weapon
2. Bruxism and Teeth Sharpening
3. The Growth and Development of Teeth for Slicing Large Chunks
4. Teeth as Weapons
5. Modern Man's Teeth are Weak Compared to Those of Primitive Man

1. Teeth are Man's Most Basic Weapon

In the human race, teeth have always been an important component of our weaponry. The information presented here explains man's basic instinct for survival through the use of our oldest and most natural means of self-defense— our teeth and jaws.

Mortal Combat is the term applied to violence associated with life and death struggles. During Mortal Combat, there are moments when the teeth are often the ONLY available and effective weapon that can provide distraction, inflict injury, and even cause death. Teeth can inflict mortal injury when applied to the exposed vital anatomy of the trachea (windpipe) and jugular vein. Teeth are also used to inflict serious injury during sexual attacks such as rape or child abuse, sometimes leading to homicide. In these cases, the assailant uses the bite as an expression of dominance, rage, and bestial insanity. And all too often teeth may be the last, or— only, line of defense in case of attack. Wise is the dentist who recognizes your teeth as such effective weaponry and he might do well to offer you dental treatment options that enhance your teeth for times of Mortal Combat.

Today, one would be hard pressed to find a martial arts school that covers the usage of teeth in Mortal Combat. One might question the necessity of teaching something that is basically a hardwired instinctive reflex. The answer is that the average person has had his/her energy pathway to the teeth and jaw blocked in some way and to some degree. This handicap inhibits the resourceful utilization of the *"dental fright/flight response"* involving the use of teeth and jaw. The possible causes of this energetic disturbance will be covered shortly. But first, a discussion about a side effect of energy restriction in the human bite instinct—Bruxism.

2. Bruxism and Teeth Sharpening

Bruxism is an involuntary, non-functional, rhythmic gnashing, grinding, and clenching of teeth—not including chewing movements—of the mandible. It is a subconscious, parafunctional condition that occurs either during stage 2 sleep or while awake. It may be secondary to anxiety, tension, or dental problems due to stress or drugs.

Bruxism activity occurs in most humans at some time in their lives. The prevalence of clenching is reported to be twenty percent, whereas sleep grinding is seen in six percent of the adult general population. It often leads to loss of tooth enamel surface, cracking of teeth, headaches, mouth and facial pain, jaw pain, and limited jaw movement.

The cause of bruxism is not completely agreed upon. Today, the general consensus among dentists is that bruxism is a pathological process intrinsically related to the dentition and/or musculature of the head and neck. If the teeth are not positioned correctly (malocclusion), the pointed anatomical cusps interfere with normal jaw movement. During function, the muscles of mastication overwork to compensate for the interferences. The muscular tension that results will eventually cause or contribute to:

- Earache
- Insomnia
- Headache
- Tooth pain
- Depression
- TMJ joint pain
- Eating disorders
- Sore or painful jaw
- Head and neck muscle pain
- Anxiety, stress, and tension

Daily stress may also trigger bruxism dependent on the level of stress, diet, sleep habits, posture, and the ability to relax. Once again, stress related muscle activation and overuse is intrinsically causal for the jaws to clench and grind the teeth

The relation of bruxism to the theory of thegosis is quite interesting. *Thegosis (meaning to whet or sharpen) describes the sharpening of anterior teeth under specific conditions, some of which may be related to social situations.* Dr. Ronald Every introduced thegosis in the 1960's to prove that bruxism is a sociological pathology. This means that a psycho-emotional driven solution rather than a physical dental/

muscular cure must be examined. He presented good evidence that primitive man's behavioral trait of clenching to strengthen jaw muscles, and grinding to sharpen teeth for self-defense, may be the basis of clinical teeth grinding.

Most dentists today treat bruxism from a physical dental/muscular direction and prescribe palliative measures to help relax the spastic muscles involved. The treatment involves a physical device such as a night guard or bite splint. This may be accompanied by massage, chiropractic manipulation, biofeedback, hot-cold therapy, far infrared light, acupuncture, acupressure, hypnosis, nutrition, herbs, etc.

Very few dental professionals accept or treat bruxism as a psychosocial pathology. Dr. Every was not able to win many supporters for his theory of thegosis, even though he spent over thirty years analyzing and presenting convincing historical data to the scientific world. I believe part of the obstacle to the acceptance of his ideas is the fact that dentists choose their profession because they like to work with their hands. They love drilling, bridging, implanting, broaching, rotor-rooting, root canaling, grafting, carving, shaping, brushing, painting, etching, bonding, slathering, smoothing, polishing, and glossing teeth. Ask a dentist to sit down and talk about emotional psychosocial pathology in relation to bruxism, and be prepared for blank stares as he hides his furious and desperately twisting fingers from your vision, constructing a midair dream of his next patient's fixed cosmetic enhancement.

Thegosis would likely be more accepted if dentists could be convinced of the benefits in connecting with their own life force/chi, and then, through that lens, using their chi to examine the source of bruxism. Once one establishes one's own reconnection of chi to the teeth and jaws, connecting the dots from bruxism to muscle building and teeth sharpening is mere child's play.

Paleontologists may never find enough convincing evidence of teeth sharpening in humans, but the chi never lies about the past. We need only interpret the results of our own investigation with wisdom and maturity.

This is my challenge to all dentists: *Let us connect with our chi, come to know and understand it, and use it to help our patients overcome their patterns of disease and pathology simultaneously on all levels—physical, mental, and spiritual.*

3. The Growth and Development of Teeth for Slicing Large Chunks

Dr. Every defined thegosis as *"sharpening a tooth, beak or bill by deliberately and forcefully grinding it across surfaces of an opposing tooth, beak or bill."* It is used by many vertebrate and invertebrate animals in order to sharpen the teeth for use as tools and/or weapons. Some examples are:

- Rat
- Sheep
- Baboon
- Sea urchin
- Vampire bat
- Hippopotamus

Dr. Every theorized that humans grind their teeth with the evolutionary purpose of honing the incisors to a sharp edge for cutting and slicing in battle. Thegosis also strengthens the primary muscles used for biting in self-defense—

the masseter and temporalis. It takes only a couple days
of clenching to rapidly pump up the biting muscle fibers,
enabling a stronger, deeper, and more lethal bite. This process is called the *"dental aspect of the fright/flight response"*
and may have enhanced the survival odds of early humans.

In order to better understand teeth sharpening within
the theory of thegosis, we should follow the growth and
development of human teeth beginning with birth.

An infant is born toothless in order to more efficiently
suckle at the mother's breast. As the child matures, the teeth
erupt to help break down solid food and this initiates the
child's eventual separation from the mother. The child must
then strengthen its muscles of mastication to begin self-
feeding at nature's table.

When an infant is born, the entire gut, including the
colon, is sterile. However, as the baby's head begins to slide
through the vagina, bacteria are picked up on the infant's
lips. When it suckles on the mother's nipple, more bacteria
are swallowed with the milk. As the baby begins to eat more
solid food, pre-chewing transfers even more bacteria to the
intestinal flora. The mother must pass to the child her own
prebiotic and probiotic bacteria necessary to digest solid
food and enhance immunity to disease. This is a normal and
desirable sequence of events.

Nature originally intended the mother to chew, soften,
and transfer predigested food to the child's mouth. This
teaches the child with newly erupting teeth to safely chew
and swallow solid food without aspirating whole particles
and choking to death. Pre-chewing food is no longer a part
of today's modern culture, but it is a practice still seen in
poor, developing countries. Why take the time to chew your

baby's food when you can buy a jar of commercially blended baby food at the local grocery store? I'm joking, of course!

Mother's milk is BY FAR the most potent source of nutrition, minerals, and vitamins for the infant. It is also the very best source of prebiotics and probiotics for the brand new bacteria factory in the baby's colon. Infant formula manufacturers have been forever trying to replicate mother's milk, but nothing comes close to what a mother's natural milk and saliva does to create a healthy environment in the baby's colon. Likewise, commercially blended baby food could NEVER replace the healthy benefits of pre-chewing.

Science has shown that the infant's health is directly affected by that of the mother, beginning with its life as an embryo. Infants who are breastfed and whose mothers consumed foods containing prebiotics or took prebiotic supplements, both before and after birth, have much fewer and less intense allergies as they mature. A natural childbirth through the vagina, in addition to breastfeeding, provides the infant with healthier gut bacterial colonization than those who are born by cesarean and are fed commercial formulas.

However, it is best to use caution if you consider pre-chewing your baby's food, as beneficial as well as harmful bacteria are transferred from mother to child. Mothers should make every effort to stay healthy in all physical and mental respects. The infant's health is affected, for better and worse, by bacteria and viruses that are passed between mother and child. Healthy vaginal and oral inoculation of the infant remains a prominent marker of good health, even into adulthood and beyond. Passing harmful bacteria and viruses can promote disease and life-threatening medical

issues even in the adult years. There has been one verified
case of a mother passing the AIDS virus to her child by pre-
chewing food. Mothers pass along as many as five hundred
different species of bacteria and viruses, including those
that cause tooth decay, gum disease, hepatitis B, hepatitis
C and Group B streptococcus, among others. If a woman is
planning on having children, she should be aware of this and
do everything possible to improve her own health before
becoming pregnant. Newborn babies deserve every chance
for a normal, healthy, disease-free life.

As previously discussed, one of the reasons humans
have teeth is to facilitate complete separation from the
mother. This is part of a logical progression and schedule, all
related to the eruption of the baby's teeth. Let's now examine the role teeth play in the theory of thegosis.

Deciduous (baby) teeth are smaller, with thinner protective enamel, and have less prominent cusp tips compared
to adult teeth. Their main purpose is help the child make
the transition from liquid breast milk to softer food solids.
Logically, the smaller mouth and less developed muscles of
the growing child influence the appropriate size and shape
of tooth to perfectly chew the next stage of soft food solids.
Baby teeth are "pint-sized" compared to full-sized adult
teeth. The baby is not yet strong enough or experienced in
safe technique to tackle hard, tough foods it would find in
its environment. It has to remain attached to the mother a
little longer. Evolution has mandated tiny baby teeth for the
child as the best size and strength for the job at hand.

At about twelve years of age, the child's deciduous teeth
have been replaced by twenty-eight fully formed adult
sized teeth. The child has become a young adult with a

larger, muscled body, and stronger, thicker, enameled teeth. Psychologically and physically the young adult is ready to freely begin feasting at nature's table. At this stage of development, the teenager is also ready to prepare for the more advanced and formidable adult task of using his/her teeth as tools and weapons.

Many children today are reaching physical and sexual maturity earlier than in the past, although emotional maturity does not seem to be following this trend. American girls in the year 1800 had their first period, on average, at about age 17. By 1900 that had dropped to 14. Now it is 12. *Some scientists attribute early physical maturation to spilled and dumped chemical hormones polluting our water and food systems. I myself have seen pre-teens with their full complement of thirty-two adult teeth, including wisdom teeth. This phenomena has come about within the past twenty-five years, whereas previously the average age for wisdom tooth eruption was between seventeen and twenty-two years of age.*

At this point, teeth sharpening needs to begin in order to help the young adult survive a long healthy life. Although the adult teeth are larger than deciduous, they still have relatively rounded incisor edges and cusp tips. The teeth, at this stage of development, need to be sharpened, and the jaw muscles bulked up, for efficient use as a tool for holding, cutting, molding, and softening clothing materials. They also need to be strengthened and sharpened for self-defense, in the Spirit of the Warrior.

More scientific information on the architecture of the tooth and how it becomes stronger with grinding, clenching, and tapping will be found in later chapters. But at this time, it is important to insist that readers of this text **must not attempt to sharpen and strengthen teeth without correct instruction and guidance.** *In other words: Don't do this at home.*

When chewing we grind, squeeze, break, cut, slice, chop, split, crack, crush, flake, stab, gash, and nick the food. Very few children today display advanced proficiency in all of these functions. I have never heard of a child under the age of twelve who can use their teeth to crack whole walnuts and chew through large bones. It takes an adult with adult teeth to demonstrate these minor achievements. When primitive man pushed his teeth beyond what was necessary for normal everyday function, as a tool and as a weapon in Mortal Combat, it required a strength and cutting edge MANY times more powerful and sharp than a child could manage. Children with baby teeth would be unable meet such advanced challenges.

I believe in the premise of thegosis, where primitive adults probably made a conscious effort to sharpen and strengthen the teeth and jaws, whereas today we brux sub-consciously. In primitive society, the conscious sharpening and clenching action would have enabled the teeth to be a more effective tool for fashioning garments and processing food during mastication. Clenching would also prepare men and women for self-defense by strengthening the muscles involved in grasping, attacking, and protecting. The process would have sharpened the incisor front teeth to allow a lethal bite.

Humans have a more complex anatomy and arrangement of teeth. We use our front incisor teeth mainly for slicing/scissoring and the posterior molars for grinding. The incisors and canine capture and/or segment the prey/food. The anatomy of the premolars and molars shows cusps that serve to puncture food; crests that connect cusps to shear; and basins which crush or grind food. Humans also have shorter canines than other primates. We can easily sharpen our incisors and make side-slicing actions (like using scissors) with our front teeth because our canines do not interfere. This slicing action allows us to take large chunks out of food, prey, and assailants during self-defense. All other primates use their canines as a piercing weapon instead because their canines' longer length restricts the ability to slice sideways and segment the food.

Most carnivores use their enlarged and blade-like carnassial (fourth upper premolar and first lower molar) teeth for shearing flesh and bone in a scissoring, slicing, chopping, or shearing manner. When a dog or cat brings the side of its head up against a bone on which it is gnawing, it is probably using its carnassials.

4. Teeth as Weapons

Combatants today seldom use their teeth in fighting, especially to separate and remove a large chunk of flesh in one action. This is called a "segmentative bite" and is unique to humans, not seen in primates. This aspect of our jaws and dentition is what gives us a powerful advantage over other animals during combat. Our incisor bite force is remarkably powerful—comparable to that of many predators—and our ability to slice sideways can cause vicious lacerations. Many of us have seen the power of human teeth and jaws as aptly demonstrated by martial artists pulling multi-ton vehicles with their teeth, and many are undoubtedly familiar with the story of the Chinese burglar who could bite through iron bars.

Examining bruxism through the lens of thegosis makes good sense to me, and I believe further research into thegotic theory is warranted. In today's world, teeth grinding and clenching during subconscious bruxism may be interpreted as the chronic result of social conditioning to suppress, or repress, instinctive aggression. Many people today are failing to deal with psychosocial and emotional stressors that perpetuate defensive behaviors. This purportedly explains why stress is such a common factor in people who experience elevated levels of bruxism, particularly at night when they are asleep and not suppressing those emotions. People feel under attack, so subconsciously sharpen their teeth to defend themselves. One can make a strong *a priori* case for human teeth being used as weapons by our earliest ancestors. Today, however, for a variety of reasons, the growth and development of our teeth and jaws for use as a weapon has been stunted.

One reason for this is man's invention of, and modern dependence on, sophisticated weaponry. The relatively non-lethal hand has become more important with the introduction of artificial weapons such as club, knife, bow, gun, etc. Emphasis on survival has been deflected from the simple instinctual use of mouth, teeth, and jaws to the more superior, complex manipulation and coordination of hand-held weapons. The "open hand" needs formal training to develop into a deadly weapon. Warriors are trained in the deadly use of hand combat to police and protect the social congregation. This kind of organizational control helps maintain the species. Today, more than ever, "closed hand" cutting-edge military weapons require advanced training in use.

Societal restrictions on the use of the hands by warriors is almost non-existent, save for eye gouging, but society does place restrictions on the use of teeth. This is because, in the untrained human, the teeth are more lethal than the hand. The use of biting to kill does not need to be taught, as everyone possesses this instinct for survival. Biting is extremely dangerous and many of our ancestors undoubtedly perished as the result of infection due to virulent oral bacterial flora acquired through biting during combat. Taboos were placed on aggressive actions with teeth in order to preserve the population and growth of the community and in order to prevent chaos, death, and depopulation. Taboos on fighting with the teeth were also put in place by ancient dictators for reasons that will be examined in later chapters.

5. Modern Man's Teeth are Weak Compared to Those of Primitive Man

We no longer have warriors who use their teeth as weapons. Our crooked teeth and relatively weak jaws are almost never used in a life and death struggle. We rarely read about a person biting in self-defense as one last desperate attempt for survival. These facts usually remain hidden in autopsy reports and the media has little stomach for printing such shocking stories. But *why* has man almost entirely ceased to use teeth as weapons?

Paleontologists have studied primitive skulls and, for the most part, all artifacts show sufficient room for the normal thirty-two tooth dentition. Bite malocclusion appears to have been rare in ancient man, whereas today bite malocclusion is common. Studies have shown that the mean bite force of children changes with the occlusion (position of the teeth in the arch). Malocclusion (crooked teeth) results in weakened bite force. This is likely another possible reason why humans today rely less on their teeth during self-defense. Some researchers investigating the record high incidences of malocclusion in children believe that genetics and environmental factors play an important role.

We know that nutrition in the foetal stage affects the determination of tooth size. Increased tooth size is related to increased consumption of protein and fat in the modern diet. Vitamin and mineral deficient diets, along with hormone disruptors found in food and water supplies, lead to smaller bone growth, including the jaw. Larger teeth and smaller, more constricted jawbones leave less space for the teeth to erupt into their correct position and results in crooked teeth and weaker biting power.

The growth of the chewing apparatus may be affected by the eating behavior of children from infancy through puberty. It is known that bottle fed babies have a weaker structure and function of the jaw biting apparatus compared to babies who are breast fed. People who eat coarsely milled staple grains have more developed jaw muscle structure than those who eat a softer diet. Another factor that affected bite force in primitive man was the clenching of teeth and chewing on twigs, leaves, gum, and meat jerky—processes that can develop the masseter muscle, the driving force for biting. People who clench and chew on hard substances develop more muscle fibers in the masseter, resulting in greater jaw strength. Because of our processed fast-food diet, we chew less and the things we chew are softer. People also do not have, or are unable to make, the time to eat at a leisurely pace and chew their food thoroughly. And the result is that modern man's biting apparatus is weak in comparison with the diamond-steel teeth and massive jaws of our ancient relatives.

Another modern phenomena that contributes to weaker dentition is the preponderance of wisdom tooth extractions. As our brains continue to evolve and enlarge, our jawbones are becoming reduced in size to make more room within the skull. Genetic and environmental factors also explain why less dependence on the teeth and jaws for daily living leads to smaller jaw bones in humans and constricted room for wisdom teeth.

I hope that I have put forth enough theory, ideas, and opinions to illustrate my premise that our teeth, *rather than our hands,* remain our most primitive and primary weapons of choice. It is almost unheard of these days for a human to aggressively or defensively bite a fatally vulnerable neck. We repress our instincts and no longer have the sharp teeth and commanding jaws that would confidently bring us victory in battle. Instead, the modern one-on-one battle between warriors usually comprises high tech hand weapons such as guns or knives.

Later chapters in this book will continue to reveal how our society artificially controls and restricts the use of teeth in their ultimate, basic, instinctive use for self-defense. Historical evidence for this tragedy is not likely to surface, and the true reasons will probably remain buried and unknown, but the effects on humankind are obvious. Solutions to correct this current deficiency in the fight for survival during mortal combat are forthcoming.

3

Return to the Source

The ancient tai chi texts exhort students to *return to the Source,* or return to the Tao, through introspection and reversal of the process of creation. This is another reference to the Taoist theory of evolution. Taoists adhere to the idea that for self-discovery one must reverse the path one has followed and discover one's true identity at the Source, understand it, be one with it. Then, using creative evolution with the mind, design a new blueprint for the future. This is a theory of the path to immortality.

The reversal starts with a meditation on your present day situation described as a "full cup of tea." Empty the cup to become pure Yin, devoid of ego, still, silent, ready to accept the knowledge that will fill your empty vessel. The meditative process will take you back to your birth experience or perhaps further, back to the womb. Beyond the womb, you may encounter our energetic connection with animals, and beyond that, eventually reach the Source. In theory, your chi is most pure and powerful at the Source. For this reason, I believe the practice of meditating on the animal forms is of vital importance to those interested in self-defense. Take your mind and chi back in time and swim within the weaving river of energy that flows from the animal kingdom. Drift and bob in its current in order to absorb the pure, supreme, original chi and return with it to the present day.

This is a huge reservoir of pure energy linked to the power of survival. In the grip of a predator, all available chi is used to fend off death. This pure chi, transferred to and stored in the teeth and jaws, fuels the ultimate in survival self-defense as all animals use the teeth and jaws in mortal combat. Those who are able to access this primal chi can expect astounding levels of advancement in their practice of martial arts. This is my discovery.

I question why the masters do not delve into this realm with their students, why such foundational techniques are not part of all core-level instruction. But no matter, I am lifting the veil of mystery, just a bit, so that you may benefit immensely. In short order, the Secret Smile of Laughing Buddha will begin to bring forth many answers to questions concerning the use of teeth and jaws in mortal combat.

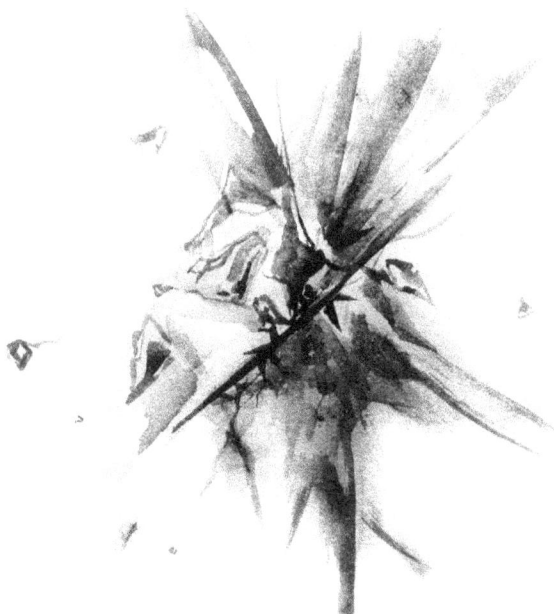

4

Diamond-Steel Teeth and Massive Jaws

For millions of years man depended upon the size and sharpness of his teeth, the bone mass density of the skull and jaws, and the biting force of the jaw muscles when defending himself, and these factors frequently decided the victor in Mortal Combat. Today we have developed superior martial art techniques and weapons of self-defense. Who needs a massive bite force? Such situations are not likely to arise as we drive to work with a double latte in one hand and a smartphone in the other.

However, if one wishes to maintain vibrant health and promote longevity, it is necessary to facilitate the uninterrupted flow of chi. Unfortunately, for many generations the oral cavity has been a blocked and neglected reservoir of original chi, and this holds true in everyday life as well as martial arts development. The average person fails to see the significance of healthy, strong teeth and jaws. People spend little time brushing their teeth in comparison to that devoted to hair styling and fingernail care. And the neglect shown to the oral cavity and surrounding physiology cannot help but have a large, negative effect on overall energy flow. It is highly unlikely that hair might play a major role in protecting your life during combat. And yes, fingernail strength has advantages, but artificial nails have no more value than cosmetic war paint. The teeth, on the other hand... it is easy to imagine the role they might play in a fight to the death.

Here are some recent discoveries that you may find interesting:

Hexagonal Diamond

Diamond is currently regarded as the hardest known material on the planet. But by considering large compressive pressures under indenters, scientists have calculated that a material called wurtzite boron nitride (w-BN) has an even greater indentation strength than diamond. And scientists have also discovered that another material, lonsdaleite—also called hexagonal diamond, because it is made of carbon and is similar to diamond—is even stronger than w-BN and fifty-eight percent stronger than diamond.

Predator X

This fifty-foot long monster is a newly discovered species of pliosaur, and researchers say the reptile ruled the Jurassic seas about one hundred and fifty million years ago. Its anatomy, physiology, and cunning all indicate that it was the ultimate predator, the most dangerous creature to stalk the deep. The forty-five ton creature propelled itself with its four flippers and relied on its crushing jaw power to take out its prey consisting of marine reptiles and fish. Predator X possessed a skull ten feet in length and a bite four times as powerful as that of T-Rex. Researchers estimate that it had 33,000 pounds per square inch (psi) of bite force. (It is interesting to note that the compressive strength of the human tooth is about 30,000 psi.) Bite estimates predict it could crush even the largest four-ton SUV.

Vegetarian Spider

Until recently, all spiders were thought to be carnivorous. A new study reveals that a vegetarian tropical jumping spider has been identified out of some forty thousand meat-eating spider species.

In the late 1800's, naturalists discovered a spider they believed to be carnivorous, but they were uncertain of its exact diet. Biologists studying the spider recently found that it eats the nutrient-rich buds of acacia plants. Also unique to this species is the manner in which it jumps from thorn to thorn in order to escape aggressive ants that live inside the hollow thorns. The spider does occasionally snack on the ant larvae, but the bulk of its diet is plants.

I included these three items because they remind us of how little we truly know, and how much we have yet to learn, of ancient history and the natural world around us. Scientists often make assumptions based on limited data that are later proven to be totally incorrect. It is in this light then that I find it easier to accept the thegotic theory stating that early man consciously sharpened his teeth. Compared to modern man, he would certainly have possessed bone-crushingly sharp teeth and jaw strength. Martial arts masters recognize that ancient man was more in touch with his primordial energy and must have kept it honed for survival. I feel certain that the chi force in primitive man's teeth and bite was incredibly superior to that of 21st century man.

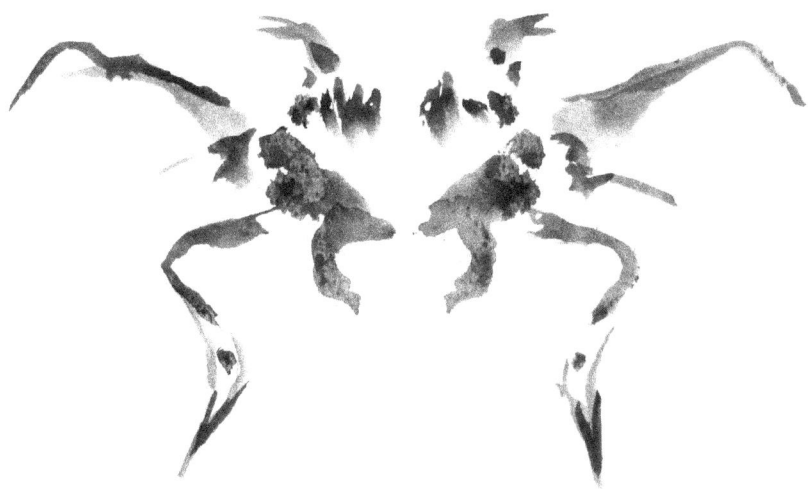

5

Human Bite Force Potential

Let's now focus on matters relating to human bite force.

A large dog can exert a bite force of up to 450 pounds per square inch.

A lion can exert a bite force up to about 1000 pounds psi.

An alligator can exert a bite force of 2000–3000 pounds psi.

The human bite force ranges from 55–280 lbs. psi—averaging 162 lbs. psi—and in some cases reaches a maximum of over 970 lbs. psi.

There is an important distinction between bite 'force' and 'pressure.' Human bite pressure has been measured at 5600 psi. However, the compressive strength, or shattering point, of a typical healthy human tooth is up to 30,000 psi. This raises an interesting question: Why do human teeth require a compressive strength of 30,000 psi if man can only produce 5600 psi of bite pressure? Is it possible that primitive man had much greater bite pressure than modern man? Did modern man lose much of his inherent strength because of changes in lifestyle? If the answer is yes, is it possible to regain our original strength, which should logically be much greater due to the 30,000 psi compressive limits of the tooth?

If it were possible to test ancient man's bite force strength and compare it to the force of today's population of relative dental cripples, the cave man would likely win.

Every time a dentist drills a tooth, the result is microscopic internal stress fractures that severely weaken resistance to compression and slowly cripple it. When a lame tooth is challenged with extreme pressure, the biter may either "give up" due to pressure sensitivity or the tooth will shatter. Take special note that a weak tooth—such as one with a large filling, internal crack, or root canal—will suffer a large loss of resistance to compressive forces and easily shatter. Ancient man rarely had serious tooth decay and so would have had no need for dental intervention. His teeth would have had more resistance to breaking and shattering than modern man's compromised tooth structure.

A tooth with an unfilled small cavity will resist compressive forces better than a tooth with a small cavity filled with mercury-silver filling. Studies indicate that a tooth with today's newer bonded white filling is more resistant to dangerous compressive forces than a tooth filled with mercury-silver. If one is undecided about the dangers of utilizing mercury-silver fillings, then this clear advantage of bonded plastic-glass over mercury-silver might be enough to tip the scales.

Twenty-first century tooth filling technology might, in some ways, give our bite force a slight advantage over that of one of our ancestors who had a small tooth cavity. Nonetheless, the person with cavities is sure to have a weaker overall body constitution than one who is free of tooth decay. This has been proven time and again, and was ably demonstrated in the past by the method of examining the teeth in order to ascertain which slaves possessed the hardier constitutions.

There is no denying the fact that mankind today, in general, is weaker in all physical aspects—including teeth and bite strength—compared to ancient populations. Recent findings have almost conclusively proven that primitive man was, by far, physically superior to modern man. Anthropologist John Mehaffey has discovered fossilized aboriginal footprints of six men chasing prey over soft muddy terrain. An analysis showed they reached speeds of twenty-three miles per hour. Today, the world's fastest man can achieve twenty-six mph. But it is highly likely that if the aboriginal men were placed on a hard, flat track and fitted with spiked running shoes, they would easily beat the current world record time. The most accurate measure of the difference in strength and ability between a cave man and a modern athlete would entail a comparison of hunting and combat skills. I would place my money on the caveman.

Other examples of physical superiority from the past: Neanderthal women had ten percent more bulk muscle than modern man. Athens employed rowers who could surpass the achievements of modern oarsmen. Roman legions marched a distance equivalent to one and a half marathons every day while carrying equipment heavier than their body weight. Photographs from the early twentieth century showed young tribal African men accomplishing standing high jumps of up to eight feet as a rite of passage.

And from a mental perspective, as martial artists, our skills and strengths are to a large extent determined by how well we can concentrate and focus our chi. There is no comparison between the shortened attention span and scattered thought processes of modern man and the intensely focused "survivalist" mind of prehistoric man. Concentration and survival are necessarily inseparable. We believe ourselves to be more intelligent, but are we really? Perhaps it is only the vast pool of past experience we have to draw upon to synthesize new data that allows us to feel more intelligent.

But our bite force is unquestionably weaker. When was the last time any of us had to crack open nuts, or crush the neck or leg of a small game animal with our teeth to access the nutritious marrow? It is just not necessary, and one of the results of our softer lifestyle is the neglect of the chi container that comprises the teeth and jaws.

If we can only begin to develop and focus the chi in our mouths to the level of our forebears, and merge this energy into the flow of our major meridians, our capacity for fighting might be restored to the magnificence that nature originally intended.

This is what I have seen in my own personal experience and why I am sharing this information that is **RARELY** discussed.

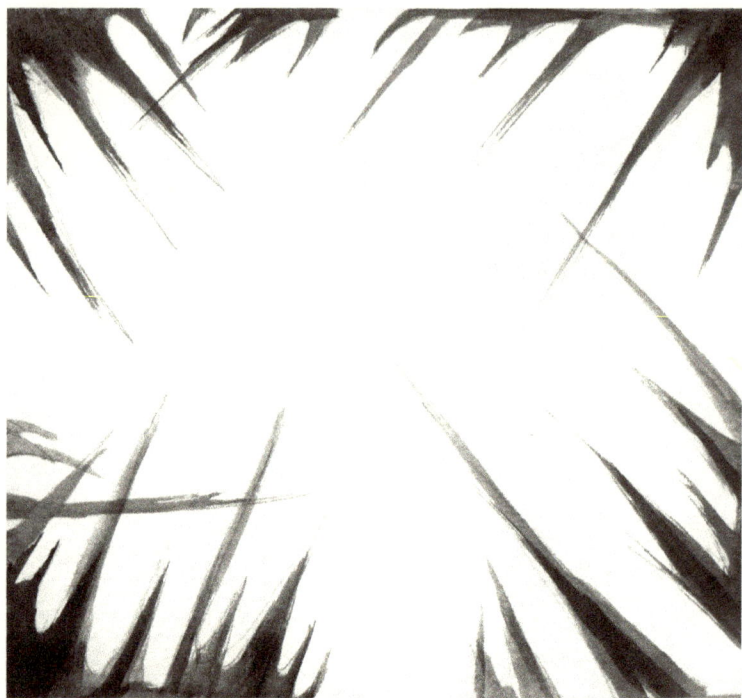

6
Biting in Sports

We know that human biting is sometimes involved in violent crimes. The average law abiding citizen, however, also occasionally unleashes the instinct to bite while actively engaged in sports. And athletes functioning at peak intensity often discard all social conformity in order to tap the deep, basic energy needed for victory. The following true events illustrate this point:

Conrad Dobler, the offensive lineman billed as "Pro Football's Dirtiest Player" on the cover of Sports Illustrated in the summer of 1977, admitted to biting Minnesota Vikings defensive tackle Doug Sutherland on the finger.

Ottawa Senators forward Jarkko Ruutu was suspended by the National Hockey League for biting an opponent during a game. Ruutu bit Buffalo Sabres enforcer Andrew Peters on his thumb. Ruutu clamped down on Peters' right glove, catching his teeth on the player's thumb, which is not padded. The force of Ruutu's bite broke the skin and drew blood. As Peters pulled away in pain, his glove was ripped off by Ruutu's bite.

Nashville Predators forward Jordin Tootoo, the pride of Nunavut, was alleged to have bitten the pinkie finger of Columbus Blue Jackets forward Tyler Wright during a game in January 2004.

A high school wrestling coach in Pennsylvania resigned after he allegedly bit one of his wrestlers in the leg during practice.

Former Sydney Swans player Peter Filandia was sus-pended for 10 matches after pleading guilty to biting an opponent's testicles during a game.

Hockey star Marc Savard was suspended for one game in 2003 when, playing for Atlanta, he bit Darcy Tucker on the glove in a game against Toronto.

New Jersey Devils forward Travis Zajac was wrestling Philadelphia Flyers defenseman Derian Hatcher after the whistle. Zajac offered a face washing to his opponent, and ended up with a bitten middle finger that required stitches.

In 2001, Sevilla midfielder Francisco Gallardo helped teammate Jose Antonio Reyes celebrate a goal by bending down and biting his penis.

In the last fifty seconds of their middleweight bout, with Adrian Dodson five rounds ahead of Alain Bonnamie on the referee's scorecard, the fighters tangled on the ropes and Bonnamie emerged with bite marks to his midriff. Dodson was immediately disqualified.

Rangers center Brandon Dubinsky required a tetanus shot after being bitten on the arm by Caps defenseman Shaone Morrison during an altercation.

And finally, the bite heard 'round the world: Mike Tyson's second fight against Evander Holyfield was stopped when Tyson bit Holyfield's ear in the third round. In a clinch with Holyfield, Tyson tore into his opponent's right ear and bit off a one inch piece of upper ear cartilage and then spit it out as the crowd was just beginning to register the shock. Tyson was penalized two points and the fight continued until he then bit Holyfield's left ear. Tyson was immediately disqualified for biting both ears. His boxing license was later revoked for this and other bad behavior. Kevin McBride, who had fought Tyson four years earlier, told one British tabloid following the famous bout with Holyfield: "Tyson is still crazy. He bit my nipple! I didn't realize it at first, but he had his teeth around it."

And here are a couple of related incidents that were not strictly sports-related:

Elizabeth Loveday was heard shouting "I'll kill you" at her ex-husband while leaving the courthouse. She then took a swing at the court-ordered marriage mediator and bit the woman on the forearm.

Investigators said a Mr. Daniel Allen, an HIV-positive resident of Clinton Township, Michigan, confiscated a foot-ball that landed on his lawn while area children and teens were playing nearby and refused to return it to the group. Winfred Fernandis, Jr. approached Allen and asked for the ball. "The suspect (Allen) went nose to nose with the victim (Fernandis) and then bit him on the mouth," said the Detective Captain. "The bite went nearly all the way through his mouth."

But in my opinion, the epic combat bite of all time occurred when David slung a stone into Goliath's eye. Then David, crouching at Goliath's giant ankle, lunged teeth first into his Achilles tendon, chomped down, and dropped Goliath like a cut tree.

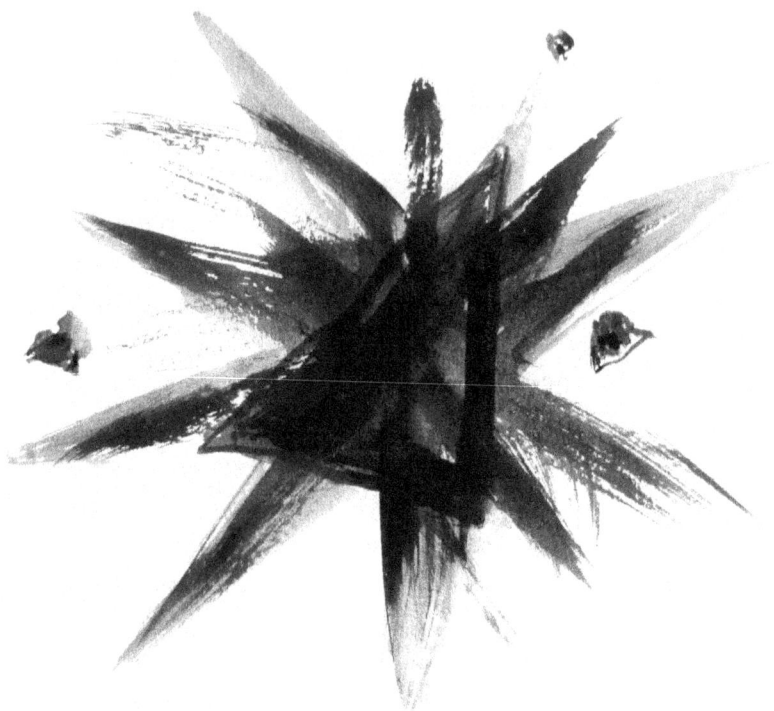

7

All About Taboos

7a The Physical and Psychological Science behind a Lethal Bite

Modern man's teeth are not shaped for puncturing, slashing, and deep penetration of tissue. Today a human bite to the throat would not likely sever any primary blood vessels, but the *pressure* of a strong bite could certainly crush the trachea and tear a blood vessel, leading to a quick death from internal bleeding and suffocation within minutes. (Death from a lethal bite to the neck in an animal usually occurs within five to ten minutes if the carotid artery or jugular vein is severed. Rapid blood loss leads to brain death.) Most martial artists today do not focus on developing the jaw and would have trouble using their teeth to put down an adversary. But in the event that they were relatively successful, the searing wound would put their opponent at a significant disadvantage and end in a slow decline in life force.

Primitive man had a much stronger bite. A deep, pressing bite to the front or side of the neck could easily cause shock, bleeding, suffocation, and paralysis leading to the death of the victim. And in ancient times the bite forces were even greater when we consider the closer connection man had to his energy. It is Intention and Chi that generate power, and during an encounter the first man to engage the throat of the other with such force would certainly be in a winning position.

Today, although the average bite of a human only ranges from 165 pounds up to 285 pounds per square inch, there have been some instances of human bite forces measured in the neighborhood of 1000 pounds per square inch. These modern fellows are much weaker than primitive cave men, so one can only imagine what tremendous bite forces ancient man achieved. A lion is capable of exerting 950 pounds of force; imagine being bitten in the throat by an opponent exploding with a lion's roar!

The anatomy of the throat and neck presents a study in contrasts. The relatively soft throat is very vulnerable to attack as a powerful bite in this area can crush the trachea (windpipe) resulting in rapid death by suffocation. The larynx (voice box) is safer as it rests too high up to be crushed by a human bite. (Primitive man had a hairy throat, which some investigators believe was useful for intimidating predators.) On the neck, the hard posterior of the cervical spine is a combination of skin, fat, fascia, muscle, tendon, ligament, bone, cartilage, blood vessels, and nerves which form a protective padding. Ancient man's short, thick, stocky, hairy neck lent further protection against human bites. It is very unlikely that a bite attack would have occurred from the rear into the cervical spine.

In a fight to the death, every weapon at hand is used. Primitive man, being free from taboos, would have certainly engaged his mighty jaws to bring down an enemy. Then, had the opening presented itself, fingers, toes, and ears would have been open to dismemberment. He would have torn at the flesh with his capable teeth to maul, maim, and rip blood vessels, eventually crushing the windpipe.

However, it is not possible to consider biting as an uncommon occurrence. Those of us with children are aware that they go through a period of imprinting their bite on other children's arms and legs. So common is this developmental behavior in children, a Google search of "child biting" displays nearly 30,000,000 possible hits. But if biting another person is such a natural part of human consciousness and behavior, why should society restrict its use with taboos?

Perhaps because when teeth are used as weapons, vicious passions are involved—those of anger, control, and destruction. One of the most notorious serial killers of the twentieth century, Ted Bundy, savagely bit his victims. During sexual attacks, women are usually bitten on the breasts, buttocks, and legs and men are primarily bitten on the arms and shoulders. These attacks are perpetrated by mentally unstable people, possessed of twisted and distorted energy.

It is easy to see in this light why taboos on biting might have arisen to prevent such aberrant behavior. But when such savagery was unleashed in self-defense against wild animals, the emotional circumstances were far different and the act of biting easily justified.

7b Exercise to Escape the Taboo on Biting in Self-Defense

There are reasons why few martial art teachers focus on the bite:

First, there are social taboos which can lead to scandal, loss of reputation, and bankruptcy if disregarded.

Second, as a weapon, there is too much deadly power packed into such a small part of the body. Very few students are emotionally ready to approach the study. Mistakes during training might result in serious physical and emotional consequences, and Masters today do not want to take on the liability involved in teaching these techniques.

Third, human nature is such that once one possesses such knowledge and power, there is a reluctance to share it. Masters keep most of these abilities close to the vest as it adds to their allure as an instructor and ensures a healthy income.

Clearly, if one wants to attain the highest levels in the martial arts, teeth and jaw development should be an important part of the training. And this training is not focused only on the physical aspects of teeth, muscle and bone, but rather strengthening the chi of the head, neck and oral cavity.

The following exercise is the first step in breaking the bondage of societal taboos:

1. Begin in the horse stance. Imagine that you have no arms, or clasp your hands behind your back.

2. Imagine you are an animal in a tug of war using your teeth. The head and neck are active while the legs remain rooted. Maintain a Zygomatic Smile. (A zygomatic (Duchenne) smile is the real thing, a genuine heartfelt smile that involves upturned corners of the mouth and wrinkling at the eyes. The brows lower and the eyes seem smaller as the muscles around the eyes contract; it is very difficult to fake or produce on demand.) If you have difficulty visualizing two lions tearing apart a carcass, see yourself as a domesticated dog playing tug-of-war with another dog for possession of a toy.

3.   When you get a good feeling for the tug, begin tak-ing steps in various directions as the tugging becomes more active.

4.   At this point, 'grow' back your arms and drop into your usual martial art form in a slow, meditative way, while continuing the tug of war. This can be difficult initially as you have to split your mind. Tai Chi teachers say the eyes lead the hands. (But if you are blind, then what?) In this case the teeth lead the hands. Wherever the teeth lead, the hands should follow, like a whip. I believe putting the whipstock between the teeth is a faster way to learn to connect move-ment with intention.

This chi-development exercise is very active, every muscle fiber in the body is cut and tensed, as if in a struggle for survival. This is not relaxed, sleepy, and dreamlike. You are not here to be hypnotized—this is **Fierce Hoopla**!

Imagination combined with physical movement will help develop the chi until it feels substantial in the mouth, head, and neck area. After a period of practice, flip into quiet breathing, swallowing, spitting, and vocalization techniques. Connect the oral flow of streaming chi to the great energy channels in the torso. Finally, this approach will make it easier to learn to swim in the Yin-Yang ocean of life.

What you have just read is suckling milk to whet your appetite. If you really want the meat, you need a Master to pre-chew the food and then transfer it to you. Without the Master's extraordinary enzymes, nature's banquet might be hard to digest.

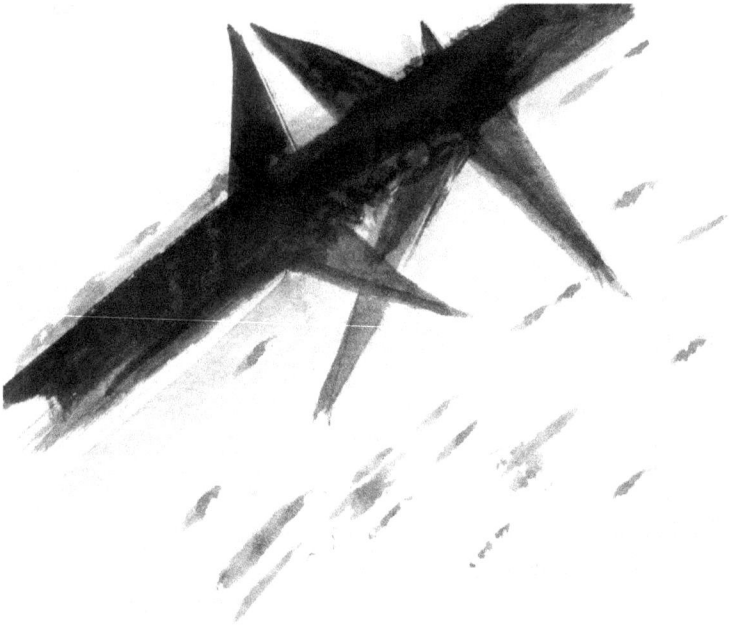

8
Anatomy of a Smile and Bite

The zygomatic smile utilizes many more facial muscles than we can easily control voluntarily. It is therefore almost impossible to fake the zygomatic smile, and most of us can immediately distinguish it from a "phony" smile. The Buddha image has been painted, engraved, and sculpted into artwork worldwide and some versions have Buddha displaying a typical zygomatic smile. This representation is known as the Jolly Laughing Buddha. In fact, some depictions show Buddha with a smile so extreme that the eyes and brows are contracted to the point where he looks *fierce*. The artist who first depicted Buddha with a fierce smile understood the qualities of a zygomatic smile. A fierce smile is what I believe to be the martial artist's perfect expression of his art. I call this *"Fierce Hoopla!"*

How are the teeth and tongue positioned during a zygomatic smile? Hearty laughter is usually vocalized with the lungs and larynx, but a hearty smile can be silent. During a silent zygomatic smile, the tongue is pressed against the roof of the mouth, the lower mandible is retruded into anatomic centric relation, muscles of mastication are activated, salivary glands secrete and the ears might even wiggle.

But there is one very important aspect of this smile that is crucial for martial artists: The inward and outward appearance of a zygomatic smile is very similar, *if not identical*, to the visual markers for the head, neck, face, teeth, tongue, and jaws during Mortal Combat. The main difference is that opposite emotions are involved. One is rooted in the joy of laughter and the other springs from savage and aggressive intent. (When you practice driving chi into your teeth and jaws, you will know you are on the right track if you express and feel the identifying markers of a zygomatic smile.)

Studies have found that men who have high testosterone levels with high levels of testosterone tend to smile less. High levels of testosterone are associated with energy, dominance, persistence, combativeness, and focused attention, all qualities that are useful in the martial arts. According to the ancient texts, however, the warrior must be in balance with his environment. So those in harmony—even men with high levels of testosterone—should find ample opportunity to flash a zygomatic smile.

Entering the zygomatic smile state will puzzle one's opponents and give one a psychological advantage. Facing an adversary with a wild facial expression that may be construed either as joy or savagery is quite disarming. This is the same confusion people experience when gazing at the Mona Lisa. Depending on where one stands when studying the portrait, Mona Lisa can appear radiant and serene from one angle and serious from another.

Scientists studied dynamic facial expressions and discovered that our eyes send mixed signals to the brain about smiles. Different cells in the retina transmit different categories of information, or "channels", to the brain. Sometimes one channel is predominant and one sees the pleasant smile, and other times that channel is overridden by another and one's perception is of a grim, determined visage.

Scientists know that the retinal cells which process dead-center vision convey information about facial expressions just as well as the cells that contribute to peripheral vision. Random noise in the path from retina to visual cortex determines whether we see a smile or not. In someone regarding a smile with dead-center vision, the retinal cells might transmit data about the smile that can be interpreted as joyful. When gazing with peripheral vision, the same smile may appear fierce. The end result is confusion, or "Fierce Hoopla," a warrior's most effective weapon.

5 Major Muscles Involved in a Zygomatic Smile

1.) *Zygomaticus major and minor.* These bilateral muscles pull up the corners of the mouth. Total number of muscles: 4.
2.) *Orbicularis oculi.* One of these muscles encircles each eye and causes 'crinkling.' Total: 2.
3.) *Levator labii superioris.* Pulls up corner of lip and nose. Bilateral. Total: 2.
4.) *Levator anguli oris.* Also helps elevate angle of mouth. Bilateral. Total: 2.
5.) *Risorius.* Pulls corner of mouth to the side. Bilateral. Total: 2.

Grand total needed for zygomatic smiling: 12.

Complete Set of Facial Muscles

Auricularis anterior (2)
Auricularis posterior (2)
Auricularis superior (2)
Buccinator (2)
Corrugator supercilii (2)

Depressor anguli oris (2)
Depressor labii inferioris (2)
Depressor septi nasi (1)
Frontalis (1)
Levator anguli oris (2)
Levator labii superioris (2)
Levator labii superioris alaeque nasi (2)
Mentalis (1)
Nasalis (2)
Orbicularis oculi (2)
Orbicularis oris (1)
Platysma (1)
Procerus (1)
Risorius (2)
Zygomaticus major (2)
Zygomaticus minor (2)

Muscles of mastication (biting and chewing)

The teeth could not occlude (come together) or disclude (separate) without the five paired muscles of mastication that make it all possible:

1.) The *Temporalis muscle* is one of three muscles that close the jaw and clench the teeth.

2.) The *Masseter muscle* is a "power stroke" muscle. Pound for pound, the masseter is the strongest muscle in the body. It therefore makes good sense to depend on the "strongest" muscle in a struggle of life and death. (Hence my premise of the importance of teeth and jaw to martial artists.)

3.) The *Medial Pterygoid muscle* elevates and orients the mandible laterally during chewing.

4.) The *Lateral Pterygoid muscle* is an important muscle responsible for drawing the jaw forward when both the right and left muscles are equally active. It also moves the lower jaw from side to side when the right or left lateral pterygoid is active separately.

5.) The *Digastric Muscle* is most responsible for opening the lower jaw.

PART TWO

"AS YIN AND YANG UNITE, ALL THINGS ARE COMPLETE ON HEAVEN AND ON EARTH."

"The Supremely Profound Principal deeply permeates all species of things but its physical form cannot be seen. It takes nourishment from emptiness and nothingness and derives its life from Nature. It penetrates the past and present and originates the various species. It operates yin and yang and starts the material force in motion. As yin and yang unite, all things are complete on Heaven and on Earth. The sky and sun rotate and the weak and strong interact. They return to their original position and thus the beginning and end are determined. Life and death succeed each other and thus the nature and the destiny are made clear. Looking up, we see the form of the heavens. Looking down, we see the condition of the earth. We examine our nature and understand our destiny. We trace our beginning and see our end....Therefore the Profound Principle is the perfection of utility."

Yang Hsiung (53 BC–18 AD)

This section examines the Yin and Yang of using the teeth in mortal combat, and all of the chapters are framed in reference to the relation of Yin and Yang. Everything may be broken down into Yin and Yang, and there are two important principles to remember when working with them: There is no such thing as pure Yin or pure Yang; there is always some Yin within Yang and some Yang within Yin. And each one is always in the process of transforming into the other.

Yin and Yang may be basically viewed in this way:

Yang:

male
active
rising
external
formless
hot, bright
stimulates
firm

Yin:

female
passive
descending
internal
has form
cold, dark
suppresses
yielding

9

The Yin and Yang of Muscle

In the following chapters I will do my humble best to explain my perception of the Yin/Yang concepts as they relate to the physiology of the face and oral cavity, and also jaw strength, chi, and bite. I feel it is important to understand and be constantly aware of these concepts if one wants to improve their martial arts skills. Let's begin with an examination of two of the strongest muscles in the human body, the masseter and the heart.

In Chinese medical theory, each internal organ is linked with a sensory organ and the heart is connected to another muscular organ, the tongue. There is an energetic pathway between the heart and the tongue, and the tongue is the extension and expression of the heart. People tend to verbalize what is in their heart. Another theory holds that the mind resides in the heart. When one realizes that the tongue, through its connection with the heart, verbalizes and expresses the ideas of the mind, it is easy to see that the harmony between the mind, heart, and tongue constitutes an intimate loving relationship. If disharmony occurs in any of the three, it may be expressed as either excessive talking or complete silence. And when the heart is in harmony, the tongue is able to differentiate different flavors. This is why a person with advancing chronic heart disease usually loses the ability to distinguish flavors in food.

Yang Muscle

The masseter muscle of the jaw is generally considered to be the strongest Yang muscle in the body, and the teeth are seen as the hardest active male energy in the mouth. (The tongue is often cited as the "strongest muscle in the body," a claim that originated as a metaphor referring to the power of speech. This claim does not correspond to any conventional definition of physical strength. However, there may be some truth to this assertion if one compares the tongue with the masseter, and it is possible to see the tongue as Yin and the masseter as Yang.)

Yin Muscle

The heart is generally considered to be the strongest Yin muscle in the body, and the tongue, as an energetic extension of the heart, is the softest active Yin energy in the mouth.

I have discovered that the tongue is actually, in some respects, stronger than the masseter. When testing the tongue and masseter in the same space, the tongue is usually dominant. (To my knowledge, there have been no formal experiments wherein the tongue and masseter have been tested in opposition to each other.) Press the tip of the tongue with as much strength as is possible against the roof of the mouth. Then, carefully bite your teeth together as hard as you can while maintaining maximum pressure with the tongue.

In my experience, the tongue muscle pressing hard against the palate seems to prevent the masseter muscle from fully contracting. So in this case the tongue is clearly the stronger of the two muscles when competing directly against the masseter. But the tongue will fatigue sooner than the masseter and within perhaps thirty seconds, the masseter will become dominant and the comparative Yin and Yang qualities of the two will have switched. This result suggests that the tongue is in need of exercise in order to increase its aerobic activity. A different result may be obtained by placing an object between the teeth, in which case the masseter is dominant.

A. Masseter

The masseter muscle is considered the "power stroke" muscle. It has a high tensile strength in pounds per square inch due to the extreme density of its muscle fibers. Its attachment origin is the inferior part of the zygomatic arch, the protruding bone just below the eye, and it inserts into the inferior part of the ramus of the mandible, or lower part of the arm of the jaw. Its absolute strength, or maximum force exerted, is the greatest of all the skeletal muscles. The muscle attachment to the jaw forms a lever which creates a strong mechanical advantage. It is a very short, dense muscle, and because of its short length, the angle of the lever creates tensile forces greater than any other mechanical (bone-to-bone) lever in the body.

When scientists study and test a particular muscle for strength, they consider three overlapping factors:_
- Physiological strength
- Neurological strength
- Mechanical strength

Western science always explains muscle strength in the context of: physiological strength (muscle size, cross sectional area, available cross-bridging, responses to training), neurological strength (the strength of the signal that tells the muscle to contract), and mechanical strength (muscle's force angle on the lever, moment arm length, joint capabilities). Each muscle is isolated and tested against these three factors in a separate container so outside interferences cannot influence the results. If you test two different muscles simultaneously in the same space, one muscle and its testing devices might affect the performance of the other muscle.

Archimedes said, "Give me a long enough lever and the right fulcrum, and I can move the earth." Of course, the power for terrestrial dislocation would have to come from Archimedes' arm, not the lever itself. A more profound definition of strength, in the case of muscles, is that the power to displace the lever begins with the mind and *intention*, which moves the chi through the muscles to the object being displaced by way of the energy meridian pathways, nerve stimulation, and blood flow.

Western science, however, cannot adequately explain 'super human strength' and usually falls back on the explanation of an adrenaline rush as the driving force behind seemingly impossible feats of strength. Adrenaline (epinephrine) is a hormone neurotransmitter, and 'adrenaline rush' refers to the activity of the adrenal gland in a fight-or-flight response when it releases adrenaline causing the muscles to perform fermentation at an increased rate, thereby increasing strength.

The theory of chi better explains the phenomenon of how little old ladies are able to lift an automobile in a split second in order to free a crushed child: adrenaline alone does not offer a convincing explanation.

The General Relativity Theory of Chi states:

Small Muscle + Focused Mind = Relatively *Big Hurt*

B. Heart

There are different aspects of muscle strength:

- *Dynamic strength* = repeated motions
- *Elastic strength* = ability to exert force quickly
- *Strength endurance* = ability to withstand fatigue

The heart is the body's strongest muscle when its strength is calculated as continuous activity without fatigue. It is the muscle that performs the largest quantity of physical work in the course of a lifetime as it work continuously, without pause. One reason this is possible is that the heart is the first organ in the body to be provided oxygen-rich blood after it has left the lungs. As oxygen-rich blood is pumped out of the heart, the majority goes to nourish the body, but some returns immediately into the coronary arteries that supply the heart. This quick return injection provides a more constant supply of highly rich oxygenated blood, and therefore the heart does not have to rely on lactic acid production for energy.

Cardiac muscle is an "involuntary muscle" and found only in the heart. It is very similar to the skeletal muscle of the masseter except in its pattern of fiber arrangement: the masseter has regular, parallel bundles but the heart has irregular, branching angles. The masseter contracts and relaxes in short intense bursts, whereas the heart sustains longer or even near-permanent contractions. Regarding these two muscles from a Yin/Yang, male/female sexual aspect, it is clear that the masseter's male, short, Yang, intense bursts in comparison with the heart's female, Yin, sustained, longer, near-permanent contractions correlate exactly with the art of love-making.

Another variation of the Yin/Yang relationship concerns muscle stimulation. The masseter, and indeed all skeletal muscles, are stimulated externally (Yang) by nerve electrical impulses. The heart cardiac muscle is stimulated internally (Yin) by regularly contracting internal pacemaker cells. All of these muscular descriptions of the heart are Yin in relation to the Yang masseter.

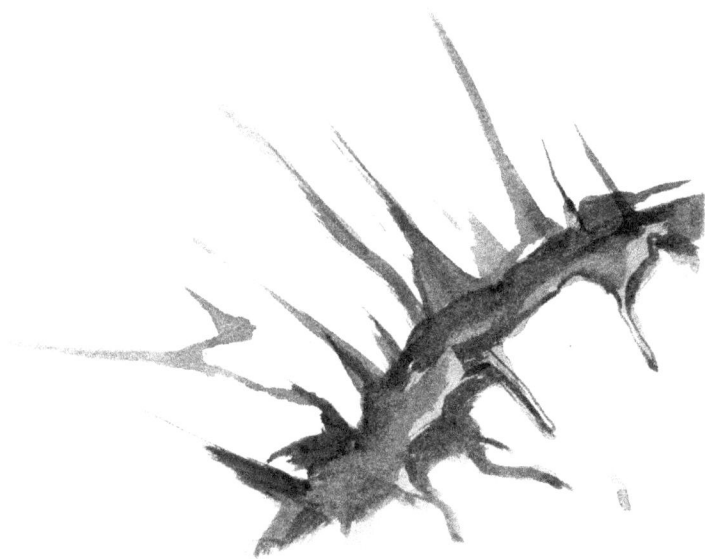

10

Tongue/Teeth

The teeth are the hardest active, male, Yang energy in the mouth and the tongue represents the softest active, female, Yin energy. In this discussion, the teeth and tongue are treated as an example of the interaction of Yin and Yang through the act of mastication (chewing food). The teeth and tongue complement each other: working in concert, they trigger the initial digestive changes in the food that we eat to nourish our bodies.

Teeth and tongue are the Yin and Yang of the masticatory system. A healthy body, mind, and spirit is in balance with all aspects of Yin and Yang. The teeth require the tongue to move and place the food onto the tooth table in order to chew food thoroughly, and the tongue cannot effectively change solid food into a perfect bolus to swallow without the help of the teeth. They must coexist in a complementary and restrictive relationship and harmonize and balance each other.

The teeth protect the tongue by setting up a nearly impenetrable 'fence' around it, and the growth and arrangement of the teeth fall under the tongue's influence. As a child's teeth erupt into the mouth, one by one, the tongue gently guides the 'fence posts' into their appropriate positions. If the child, as an infant, develops abnormal habits with the tongue (e.g. tongue thrust), then teeth develop in the wrong position and at an angle. They may protrude abnormally (buck teeth) and end up in a 'cross-bite', 'end-to-end', or constricted arrangement.

Yang tooth energy rises. This is seen in the way the teeth erupt, continually growing out of the bone socket until something impedes their movement. The body beautifully arranges this through the development of the upper and lower jaw. The upper jaw teeth grow downward and the lower teeth erupt upward until they meet and stop at just the right time and location, forming a perfect occlusion (bite) for biting, chewing, and speaking. This upward and downward eruption occurs throughout life. When a tooth is extracted, its opposite member will continue to grow and super-erupt abnormally out of its dedicated position, resulting in gum disease, tooth decay, infection, and eventual extraction of the tooth. (This illustrates the importance of the tongue's role in guiding the teeth into their correct position so they form a pristine picket fence without super-eruption.) A perfect tooth arrangement allows easy and thorough mastication of food for the most effective digestion and nutritional absorption.

The tongue consists of sixteen different muscles. It can twist, turn upside down, and bend 180 degrees, and it maintains fitness by exercising itself, pushing against the teeth and upper palate. We swallow two thousand times a day and with each swallow the tongue exercises itself by pushing upward against the palate. However, when a tooth is lost, the tongue no longer has a lateral surface to work against and it begins to lose its muscle tone in the areas where teeth are missing, becoming flaccid and swollen.

The teeth bite and chew food and utilize salivary enzymes to moisten the food into a soft, mushy state. The tongue then forms the mush into a bolus by pushing and rolling it against the upper palate. While the throat prepares to swallow the bolus, the teeth touch together one last time as the tongue goes through a wave-like motion carrying the bolus to the back of the mouth. The final act of the tongue is to pull the prepared food down into the throat where the alimentary canal is waiting to transfer it to the stomach. If the teeth and tongue cannot thoroughly masticate and prepare the food for digestion, the nutrients necessary for optimal functioning of the body will not be effectively assimilated. To a martial artist, the complementary dance between tongue and teeth is vital in a uniquely different manner, as will be shown in later chapters. And of course a well-nourished body is essential for peak performance.

Aside from the nutritive aspect, teeth and tongue also play a major role in the physical act of self-defense. The Yang energy of the teeth can easily be expressed in any number of aggressive and destructive fashions, and the tongue helps support the masseter and other muscles of mastication to provide better biting power. Whether preparing for war or in the heat of battle, a healthy, strong oral cavity is of major import.

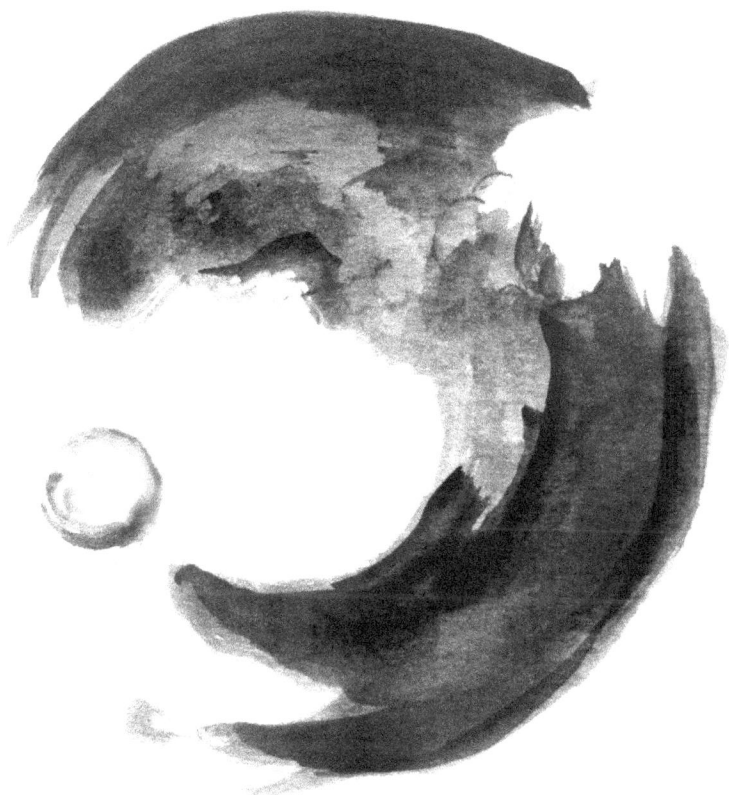

11

Passive/Active

Keeping in mind that one swallows perhaps three thousand times daily, and that with every swallow one touches the tongue to the palate, plus add in all of the speech that takes place, and it's easy to see that the tongue is a very active muscle. The teeth, however, are actually much more active than the tongue. During the waking hours of the day we are constantly tapping, biting, clenching, and grinding our teeth. In the pauses during speech, we find ourselves touching the teeth together. And at night, while we sleep, the action of teeth grinding and tapping continues. The forces exerted during night time grinding can be as great as two hundred pounds per square inch. But during sleep the tongue is passive and recovering from the day's work, even as the teeth continue to "grind through" the events of the day.

The continuous action of tapping, grinding, clenching and biting is medically termed *bruxism*. Nearly everyone in our industrial and technologically advanced countries will suffer from this condition at some time in their life. It is one of the most destructive forces wearing down the teeth, slightly ahead of acid-filled, carbonated soft drink beverages such as colas and energy boosters. Grinding is a subconscious muscle activity and most grinders grind without realizing it. The wake-up call comes when the teeth become sensitive to cold temperatures and/or chewing, one chips a tooth while sleeping or develops facial soreness. Moderate and occasional bruxism is considered necessary to resolve psychological issues that arise from day to day living, but threatens the health of the teeth and jaws if the bruxism becomes chronic, severe, and pathological.

I identify bruxism as a vibration of the teeth due to the bottom teeth rubbing against the top. Because of the hard calcium phosphate mineral structure of teeth, they also vibrate in harmonic frequency with vocal sound waves. Hard structures of the mouth, such as teeth and bone, respond more palpably to sound waves than do the soft tissue and muscle. Sound waves do travel through soft tissue, of course, making possible the medical use of ultrasound diagnostic devices. When the teeth vibrate, however, the intensity will leave no doubt that they are conducting at a greater perceptible frequency than the soft tissue. Excessive vibration initiates a protective mechanism from the tooth pulp, or center of the tooth, where vital fluids and vascular tissue (capillaries and nerves) live. The pulp's primary function is to provide nourishment to the tooth and it is, in most cases, the principle source of pain within the mouth.

As we age, the Yang teeth very clearly change size, shape, and structure. The pulp continuously creates a hard protective dentin shell. This yellow dentin lies just beneath the surface of the white enamel and, in the face of irritants, the pulp accelerates the formation of new calcified dentin as a defense, thickening the hard protective casing around the pulp. With each passing year, chronic irritation and vibration—such as clenching and grinding—thickens the dentin to the point where the pulp begins to shrink in size. Chronic irritation also stimulates the pulp to create calcified "stones" within the pulp chamber.

The Yin tongue, with its taste buds, vascular tissue and nerves, on the other hand, does not change significantly in size and structure as we age. When examining the Yin and Yang qualities of teeth and tongue, it is obvious that the teeth are far more active than the tongue. They constantly vibrate against one another in response to vocal sound frequencies from within the mouth. Environmental vibrations such as automobile traffic, human footsteps, airplane and industrial machine noises, even the quaking crust of the earth, transmit waves through the soles of the feet into the bones of the human skeleton and upward directly into the teeth. Teeth also "jiggle" with the arterial pulse, and the blood pressure from surrounding capillaries constantly pumps and thrusts the tooth in and out of the bone socket. The teeth are clearly more active/Yang than the comparatively passive/Yin tongue.

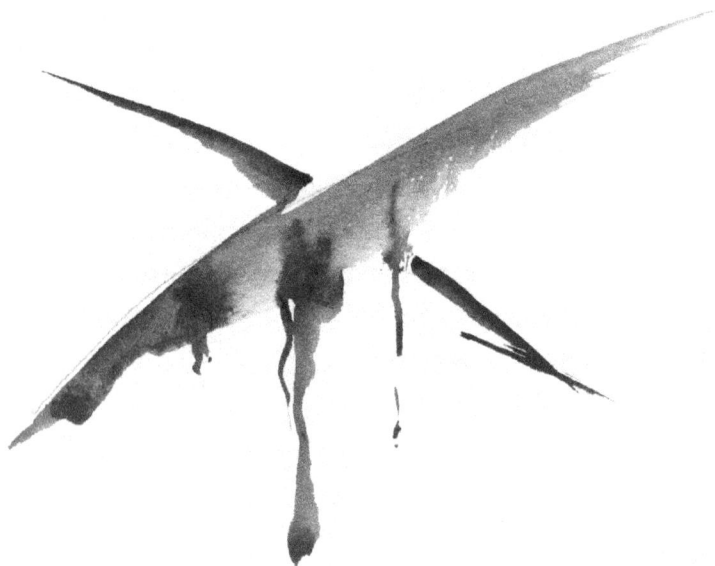

12

The Yin and Yang of Chewing and Swallowing

The digestive system is a continuous tube-like structure measuring about forty feet in length from the mouth to the anus that is designed to transport and transform solids and liquids, rendering them suitable for absorption and excretion. The teeth and tongue, together with salivary enzymes, prepare food for digestion by physically grinding it and breaking it down into small pieces to begin the digestive process. The teeth cut and grind the food and the tongue assists in moving it around during chewing and swallowing. During the process, proteins unwind so they can be separated into their component amino acids, thereby breaking the food into molecular pieces that your body can use for nourishment.

The food is then swallowed due to two types of muscle function: the first is voluntary and involves the tongue lifting the food bolus upward and backward until it reaches the back of the throat, at which point all actions become involuntary, meaning that they occur outside of one's conscious control. During the first of a series of involuntary phases, muscles move the food down and back into the esophagus to the point where the food is actively moved through the esophagus to the stomach. This action occurs through coordinated movements by constrictor muscles lining the esophagus and is not the result of gravity.

There is a definite Yin/Yang relationship between the teeth and tongue during the act of chewing and swallowing. The teeth and masseter exert an average force of twenty to thirty pounds psi on the back molars while the tongue pushes upwards against the palate with a force of about four pounds psi. In the process of rendering the food small enough to swallow, the teeth represent the greater Yang force and the tongue may be seen as lesser Yin.

To use an overly simplified analogy, the mouth is grossly similar to a nuclear reactor wherein fission releases energy. Nuclear fission is a nuclear reaction in which a heavy nucleus (Yin) such as uranium splits into two lighter nuclei (Yang), releasing energy as it does. One can say the lighter nuclei rise with the release of energy and rising is a Yang characteristic. It is easy to see the similarities between fission and mastication: the teeth break up the dense food (Yin) into lighter particles that release energy (Yang) during the digestive process. Ideally, mastication should continue until the heavy Yin particles of food are transformed into a Yin fluid ready for transport downward to the stomach. The teeth, therefore, function to release Yang energy from solid food (smaller particles) while transforming the food into a liquid (Yin) component. Conversely, the tongue takes the broken, lighter Yang food particles and passes them downward to the esophagus for their descent into the stomach, thus demonstrating the tongue's descending Yin characteristic.

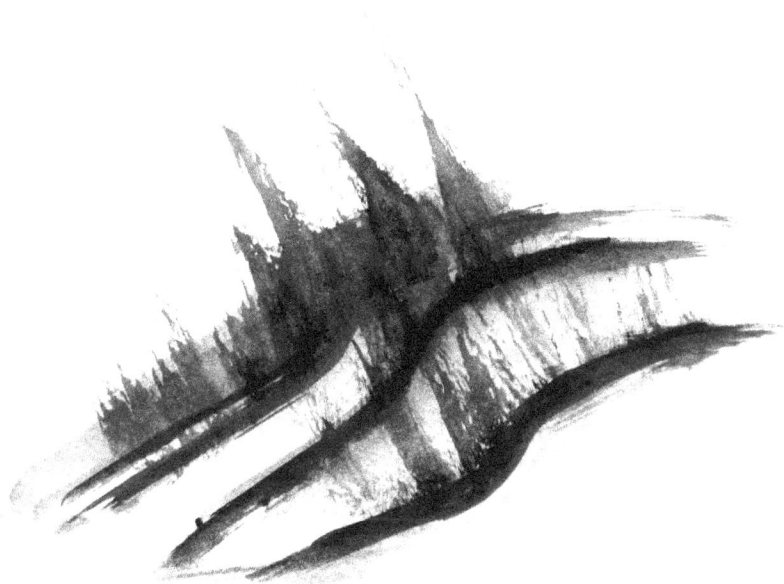

13

The Ins and Outs of the GI Tract and Why Two Natural Sets of Teeth is Not Enough

The GI tract, or alimentary canal, is a passageway for food to be transported, absorbed, and released, thereby serving as the body's food processing plant. Thirty to forty feet long from esophagus to anus, it is a muscular, extended, and convoluted tube that is actually connected with the external skin. Digestion begins at the mouth where food is chewed and mixed with saliva, adding moisture containing the enzyme amylase, which is necessary to begin to break down starches. The tongue molds the food into a ball mass known as the bolus. The bolus travels down the esophagus and through the pharynx by a muscular contraction called the peristaltic movement.

Once the bolus enters the stomach, the hormone gastrin arouses the secretion of acidic juices which further aid in the digestion of the food mass. After the stomach carries out its role in the digestive process, the food is no longer in a solid state, but has now been reduced to a liquid called chyme. The chyme travels into the small intestine to the duodenum where most of the digestive process occurs as different enzymes are released by the pancreas and glands in the intestinal wall to disassociate each molecule.

At the end of this process, each complex molecule has been broken down into its simple state. For example, carbohydrates are broken down into simple sugars, proteins into amino acids, and fats into glycerol and fatty acids. These substances are absorbed and utilized for the proper functioning of the human body. Substances that cannot be broken down by the body pass through the large intestine where the last of the water, ions, and salts are reabsorbed and the remaining solid material, called feces, is expelled through the anus.

The teeth and tongue are the gateway into the GI tract. Both arise from embryonic epithelial cells connected to skin cells and, as such, are considered to be "outside" of the body. The tongue, however, is deeper inside (Yin) the canal and the teeth are more external (Yang).

Many of us have learned, thanks to childhood trauma, that teeth avulse, or are torn out, pretty easily. The phrase "harder than pulling teeth" is widely misunderstood by the public. Pulling teeth is actually very simple if the root shape and surrounding bone density does not interfere: young conical roots with thin cortical bone plate actually extract with very little effort, and an elbow or fist to the mouth is more than enough to readily loosen and remove most teeth. The mature tooth is connected to the body by a network of fragile, hair-like periodontal ligaments which tear easily when sufficient lateral force is applied to the tooth, leaving it floating in the bone socket.

The reason for this is that the vertebrate mammal, especially the human, has teeth that have developed as expendable appendages. This expendable nature of teeth is considered a Yang characteristic. The embryo creates a tooth bud from stem cells, which, after flowering into a tooth, will eventually drop from the stem or mandible (jaw bone). The process occurs only twice in most people's lifetimes, resulting in one set of twenty baby teeth and one set of thirty-two adult teeth.

The tongue is a permanent appendage and is therefore regarded as being Yin because of that and due to its more internal relationship to Yang teeth. The anatomy of the tongue makes it impossible to tear away from its deep mounting as it is firmly attached to the body by thick muscle fibers and a vast network of nerves. The body of the tongue is made up of muscles covered by lingual mucous membranes and it is anchored to the floor of the mouth and at the rear by muscles attached to a spiny outgrowth at the base of the skull. More specifically, the muscles are attached to the lower jaw and to the hyoid bone (a small, U-shaped bone which lies deep in the muscles at the back of the tongue) above the larynx.

One major concern regarding teeth is their endurance and how to maintain their health throughout a normal human lifespan. People today in the industrialized nations live on average almost eighty years, or twice the life-span usually associated with our ancestors throughout history. An American at the time of the Revolutionary War could expect to live thirty-five years, and it was rare for people to survive much past that age. George Washington was an exception: he managed to live sixty-seven years, but late in life he required dentures. Most people in that era had poor oral hygiene and also were afflicted with the destructive habit of bruxism, making it almost impossible for teeth to endure past fifty-five years of age. In the modern world, teeth can withstand about forty years of neglect before either falling out or needing to be removed due to disease.

Scientific data seem to indicate that the human body is 'designed' to last for one hundred and fifty years and possibly as long as two hundred and fifty years. I believe human beings are probably capable of expressing a third tooth bud for a third set of teeth that would enable us to masticate well into our third century of life. It does not make sense that Mother Nature would fail to supply us with sufficient teeth to see us through our natural lifetime. Evidence for a natural second set of adult teeth does not exist, but the premise is sound. In my dental practice, I have seen many examples of relatively healthy people ninety years old—and even older— who still sport a full set of hardy, beautiful teeth. Should they remain otherwise healthy, there is no reason that their teeth should not serve them well for another sixty years; I am convinced of this certainty.

According to my theory, a set of healthy, well-formed adult teeth should endure for one hundred and twenty years in a person of otherwise exceptional good health. Accepting the possibility of the existence of a third tooth bud, then that would mathematically allow for the possibility of a two hundred and fifty year human life span: 12 years (baby teeth) + 120 years (1st set of adult teeth) + 120 years (second set of adult teeth) = 252 years total. I have no doubt that we will soon have proof of this theory's validity. We need only discover whether the trigger for a second set of adult teeth has been lost in the human genome or, if it still exists, how to naturally reestablish it.

Non-mammalian vertebrates form teeth repeatedly through a process very similar to the mechanisms humans have for replacing hair. Why do we lack this process in regard to teeth, yet retain it in regard to hair? Scientists searching for the answers to such questions may one day soon be able to grow new teeth by utilizing adult stem cells. But scientific intervention is not necessary according to my theory: if we follow nature's laws for good health, our stem cells will naturally awaken at the proper time to form the tooth buds for a third set of teeth.

14

Form/Formless

A tooth whose congenital and/or permanent external shape is changed through insult or injury, cannot regrow to its original shape. If one chips or breaks a tooth, there is no mechanism within it or the body that will heal and return it to its previous normal and functional state and shape. Scientists are currently developing ways to re-grow human enamel and are able now to regenerate an entirely new tooth. No one at the time of this writing, however, has shown that the tooth can be recreated into an exact reproduction of the original. After serious insult, the energetic memory, or blueprint, of a tooth is lost and I consider it to become formless.

The tip of the tongue, on the other hand, after suffering severe damage can regenerate to its original form. The energetic memory is contained primarily within the intrinsic muscles that actually allow the tongue to regenerate and grow back into its original shape and structure. Unfortunately, if it is damaged too far back in its body, the regenerative properties begin to decrease and it may become unable to fully redevelop. The tongue, therefore, possesses a limited memory blueprint from which it can reproduce itself. The tongue, after serious injury, is considered to retain its form for this reason.

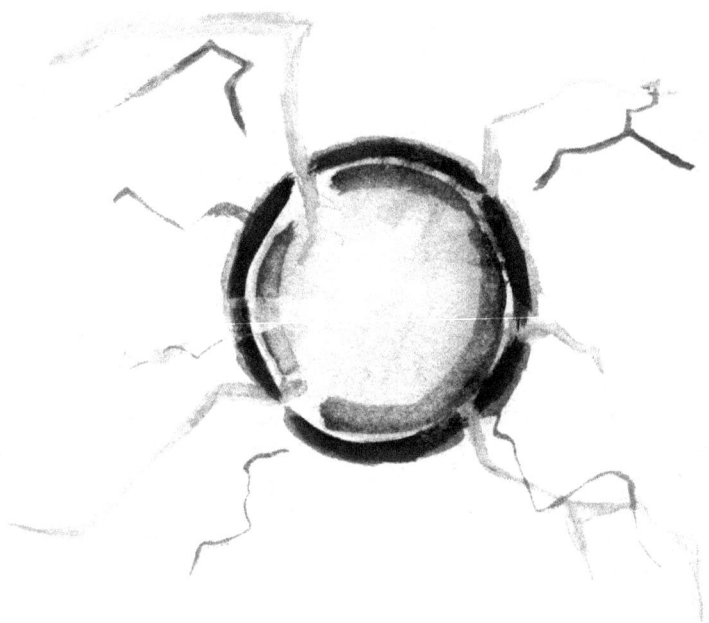

15

Pulp Friction

There are two basic components to powerful chewing and biting forces. First, there are the "chompers," or the teeth and muscles—mainly the masseters—used for mastication. The chompers cut, tear, break, grind, and mash the food. And the second component is the tongue, which is in charge of moving the food along the thirty-two tooth arches in order for every bite of food to be thoroughly "chomped." The tongue muscles develop before the masticatory muscles and the tongue's growth is completed by birth. The masticatory muscles develop later and are still not complete at birth. The teeth develop even later: the third molar wisdom tooth crown is completed between twelve and sixteen years of age.

Consider the embryonic stages of growth and see Yang as hot and developing, and Yin as cold and complete or not-developing. The teeth and masseters are seen as Yang/Hot because they continue to develop until the adolescent years, in contrast to the Yin/Cold tongue which ceases developing embryonically by birth.

The walls of the blood vessels within the tooth pulp are of necessity very thin because the pulp is protected by a hard, unyielding sheath of dentin. The dense capillary network just beneath the dentin is known for its rapid blood flow and extremely high blood pressure. Toothaches occur when the swelling pressure of an inflamed pulp has nowhere to expand and release within the constricted encasement of

the hard enamel-dentin crown. All of these features consti-
tute a Yang/Hot environment. With age, however, the tooth
pulp becomes less cellular and ultimately more fibrous leading to an overall reduction in volume due to the continued
deposition of dentin. These natural changes are all signs of
aging, or Yang becoming Yin.

The tongue's blood vessels, in comparison, exist within
the spacious compartment of the tongue and mouth. Its
vasculature does not suffer from heat symptoms as does
the compressed pulp. The tongue and its blood vessels are
cooler, more Yin and free to move within the mouth, unlike
the tooth pulp which remains caged within a hot, enamel-
dentin crown. As the body grows older, the tongue remains
cooler within its more spacious environment and appears
to age less than the teeth, which all constitutes even more
evidence that the teeth are Yang/Hot and the tongue is relatively Yin/Cold within the functioning oral cavity.

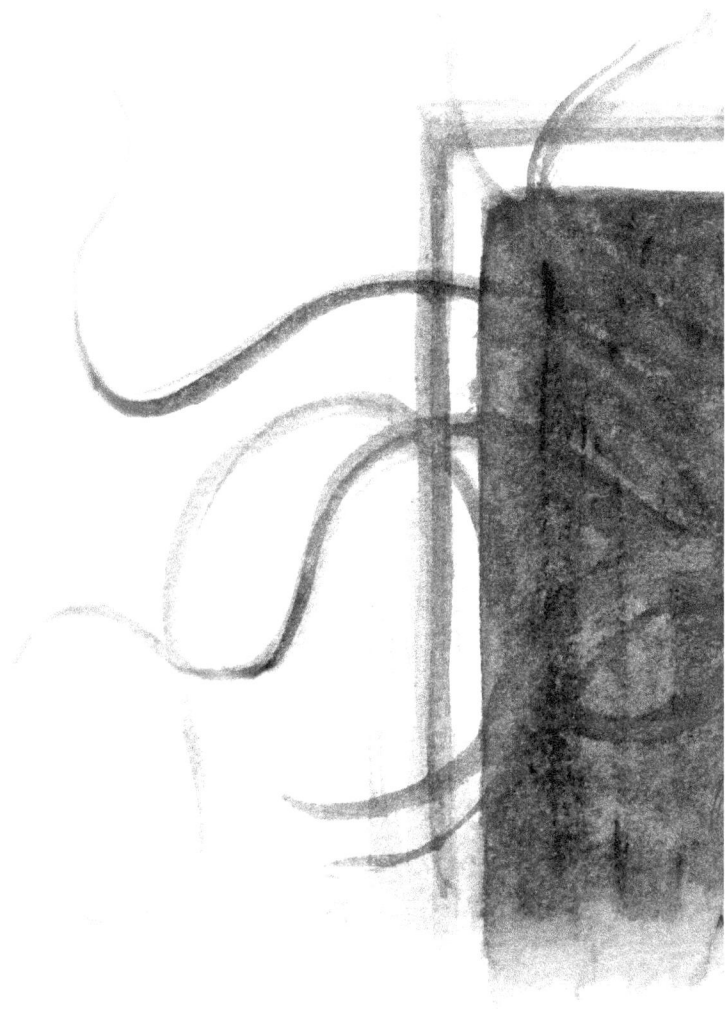

16

Firm/Yielding

Anyone who has ever accidentally bitten their tongue is intimately familiar with its yielding nature. In less than a millisecond it snaps back away from the offending tooth. Teeth, however, are relatively firm and unyielding in their attachment within the bone socket. A tooth barely senses that it is about to chomp into the soft tongue and it requires a hard bone, seed, or nut shell to send a clear message that there is a problem. And because teeth do not yield in any significant manner, they must therefore send this message to the brain, where it is further relayed to the masseter, to cease the action of biting. The masseter relaxes and then awaits further instructions before contracting again. After generating a few descriptive cuss words *and tears,* the brain rewires the pathways and allows the masseter to resume chewing.

Teeth literally hang by a threaded mesh of tangled ligaments within bone sockets and do not yield easily without the assistance of the reflex response of the motor units of the five pairs of muscles of mastication. This slight yielding nature of the tooth is mostly dependant upon the immediate inhibition response of the masseter muscle, but the tooth may also yield in a very minimal way through its periodontal attachment to the bone. It is precisely due to the fact that teeth do not readily yield that a high impact force can easily knock one out.

Studies have shown that stimulating the teeth evokes either a facilitating (boosting) or inhibiting (stopping) reflex response in the masseter. A **slow push** on a tooth will result in exciting and facilitating the masseters to contract, while a **brisk tap** on the tooth will elicit a significant reflex inhibition, or cessation of the biting action. Inhibition of the jaw-closing muscles tends to protect the teeth when one bites unexpectedly on a hard object while chewing.

The tongue, however, yields directly to unpleasant forces and does not have to rely on other muscles to protect itself. It is also capable of retracting, which is a yielding, or Yin, action. The tongue plays a valuable role in other yielding actions such as blowing bubbles with bubble gum, and whistling.

Teeth are firm and unyielding and therefore prone to chips, fractures and breaks—all Yang characteristics. The tongue is yielding and Yin.

PART THREE

AWAKENING THE BEAST OF FIERCE HOOPLA

17

Buddha Tooth

Legend has it that when the Buddha died his body was cremated in a sandalwood pyre and his left canine tooth was retrieved from the funeral pyre by Arahat Khema. A belief grew that whoever possessed the sacred tooth relic had a divine right to rule that land. Today there are at least four separate countries claiming to possess one of Buddha's teeth: according to the Chinese Government, historical texts show that only two relics exist, one held in Beijing and the other in Sri Lanka. Buddhists in India and Singapore, however, also lay claim to Buddha tooth relics. Whether these relics are authentic or not makes for interesting conversation over coffee or tea, but I wonder—what was the original reason that one of Buddha's teeth was held in such reverence?

'Buddha' translates as 'Awakened One', or someone who has awakened from the sleep of ignorance and sees things as they really are. A Buddha is one who is completely free of all faults and mental obstructions. I am not personally enlightened enough in the tenets of Buddhism, or in the details of the life of the Buddha, to discuss these matters in depth. I am curious, however, about one aspect of the many carvings, statues, portraits and other depictions of the Buddha. Why is he sometimes depicted with a large smile, and at other times with no smile? And what about *the teeth behind the smile* that is portrayed in so many images?

Interestingly, the first known images of Buddha depicted him without a smile.

The jolly "Laughing Buddha" smile is, without doubt, my favorite, and it is the epitome of a true zygomatic smile. In China, he is known as the Loving, or Friendly, One and is said to have been based on an eccentric Chinese Ch'an (Zen) monk who lived over one thousand years ago. His large protruding stomach and jolly smile have given him the common designation "Laughing Buddha", and he is known as a deity of contentment and abundance. According to legend, if one rubs the Laughing Buddha's great belly, it brings forth wealth, good luck, and prosperity.

All forms of portraits have been long regarded as high art and, at its best and most sublime, portrait painting has been considered with an almost reverential admiration. Historically, the portrait subject patiently endured a two-hour sitting and would not have been inclined to attempt to hold a definite expression of any kind, nor would the painter have thought of making such a request. A serious expression on the face of the subject was typical of fine portraits, and lightness of mood was seldom expressed in portraiture. This constraint led to the tendency for portraits to be composed, restrained, and even dignified. And throughout history, portraits have never depicted the teeth in a smile. The most famous smile, that of the Mona Lisa, is a perfect example.

It was not until the age of photography that teeth became an important component of the smile. Today's standard is a broad, toothy smile, and white teeth are crucial in creating a successful image. Yellow, stained teeth are never found in the portfolios of famous people. And according to recent surveys, yellow teeth are a major turn-off during the act of making love. The portrait smile still remains a point of contention, but the current trend tends toward naturalness and you will see more lighthearted expressions represented today than in the past.

My interest in the visage of saintly figures such as Buddha, Jesus, Muhammad, Zoroaster, and Socrates lies in the deeper core meaning. Are there secrets to be revealed behind the smile/no smile, behind broad, smiling exposed teeth? What is the meaning of teeth hidden behind closed lips? Is there more to explore and understand than what history has written?

So be it. Allow me to plant seeds in your mind that may blossom into food for thought as you journey along your Path.

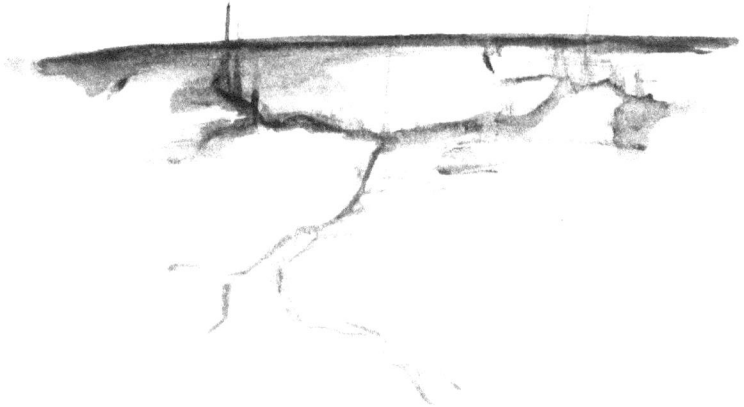

18

The Teeth and Tongue of Life and Death

To study the teeth and tongue, in my opinion, is to study a microcosm of Life and Death. First, let us examine the role of the tongue. All human instinctual drives link with the tongue. Infants use the tongue for drawing nourishment from the mother's breast. Babies use the "tongue reflex," which pushes out any foreign food or substance, to protect against choking before they are old enough to digest solid food. In a manner of speaking, the tongue reflex is the FIRST instinctive self-defense skill a human being uses to preserve its life. In adults, the tongue also plays a part in propagating life: its use in foreplay leads to procreation.

The tongue directs the ideal placement of the erupting teeth within the arches. And after the teeth begin to erupt, the baby is, in effect, taking greater charge of its destiny as the teeth become its second weapon used to defend against real and/or imagined threats. Babies and young children bite vulnerable body parts to gain needed attention and ward off unfamiliar threats in order to preserve life. It is easy to see how teeth give and take life: they masticate and soften food into a liquid state, readying the nutritive potential for digestion, and their bite forces thwart imminent danger to life. But it is the tongue, with its ability to form words that are potentially more devastating than any WMD, that is truly man's ULTIMATE WEAPON.

The teeth and tongue play an important role in balancing the Yin and Yang of the entire body. When the tip of the tongue touches the roof of the mouth, it connects two major energy pathways of the body—the Governing and Conception vessels. And when the teeth of the upper and lower jaws are touching, it contributes secondarily to connecting the two energy channels. The Governing Vessel is the confluence of all the Yang channels, over which it is said to "govern," and it is also known as the "Sea of Yang." This is due to its location and pathway because it flows up the midline of the back—a Yang area of the body—and over the top of the head and down to the upper palate. It may be used to increase the Yang energy of the body. The Conception Vessel, or "Sea of Yin," plays a major role in Qi circulation and monitoring and directing all of the Yin channels. It connects with the lower palate, and by joining the two channels with tongue and teeth in the oral cavity, Yin and Yang may be balanced throughout the body.

The teeth and tongue have a beautiful, symbiotic relationship: the tongue gently rubs, cleanses, and massages the teeth, and the teeth—the hardest substance in the body—create an almost impenetrable barrier protecting the tongue. Each supports the other, and neither can fully exist without its complement. Nature designed the teeth and tongue to last a lifetime. In the case of teeth, at least three sets are needed to serve the body until the age of two hundred and fifty years is reached. The tongue never wears out. Through knowledge of the tooth and tongue, life and death become more meaningful.

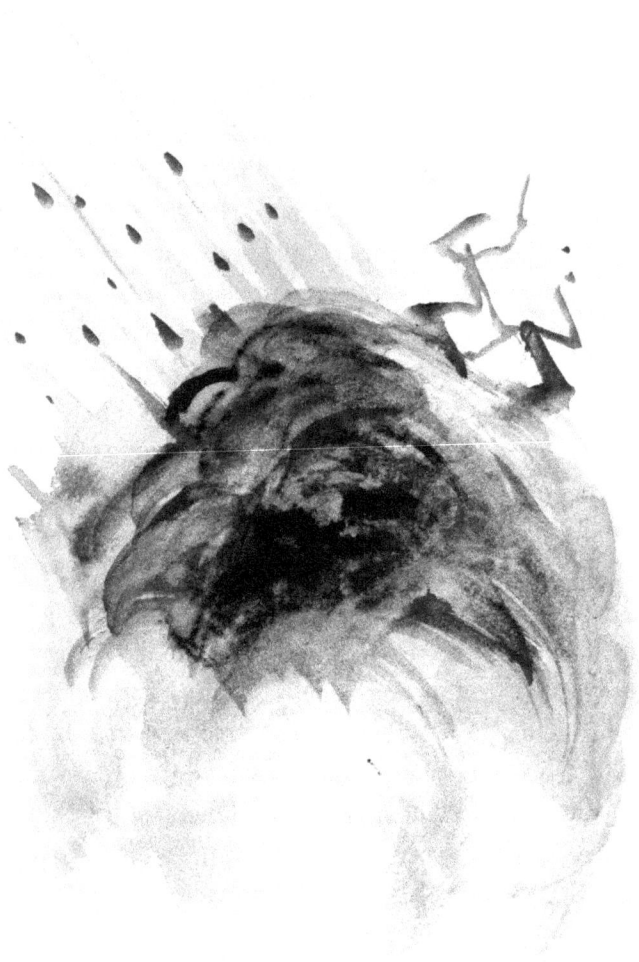

19

The Missing Link

Anthropologists searching for the missing link to our original ancestor discovered an ape skeleton in Ethiopia in 1994. This revolutionary finding reinforces the theory that chimps and humans evolved separately from a common ancestor. Our oldest known human ancestor to date, named 'Ardi' by her discoverers, roamed the forests of Africa over four million years ago. She was short, hairy, and had long arms and—similar to today's humans—stubby upper canine teeth. This is significant because scientists previously believed that our common ancestor would prove to be more chimp-like—and chimps possess long, sharp canine teeth.

The assumption exists that because Ardi's canine teeth are smaller than those in chimps and apes, this hominid species did not use them to fight and compete for mates. I believe a vital piece of information was left out of the reasoning that led to that conclusion, and the missing link in this string of logic is *chi.* Anthropologists are not knowledgeable about human energy and I feel that this shortcoming has led to a misrepresentation of the relics. Just because Ardi's canine teeth are not as long and sharp as those of chimps should have NO bearing on their use for fighting and competing for mates.

Contrary to popular belief, size and shape is not every-thing and I do not believe that a stubbier canine tooth is less effective in mortal combat than a long sharp one, or that the longer, sharper version guarantees success. Every variety of tooth shape and size possesses *Chi Potential.* Combatants must necessarily utilize all of their tools—without focusing on any perceived disadvantages or advantages—to the fullest extent in order to triumph. And the focus should be on how to bring out the full potential of the teeth by refining the chi. Believe me, if teeth are possessed of refined chi to the extent that they can bite through iron, the shape and size are irrelevant. The person who can develop and use their chi will ultimately win the fight over another who relies only on the physical.

At this juncture of my dissertation, it is time to focus on biting during mortal combat. This chapter is the missing link for the development of chi in the jaw muscles, bones, and teeth. All that has come before—from the Buddha's smile, Yin-Yang properties, Ardi, Predator-X, to disagreements about the importance of size and function—merely constitutes a simply chewed meal, the relevance of which is to illuminate the possibility of something beyond the obvious. But when the goal is developing martial arts skills, one must bite hard and deep into the hide.

In order to take another step forward in your understanding of energy within the martial arts, focus on the teeth and tongue. Every part of the body connects to and benefits the whole, and the teeth and tongue are no less important than the foot and fist when in combat. They may, however, be a missing link in your quest to understand chi and chi potential. It is necessary to use imagination, visualization, and a deep understanding of your inner feelings in order to discover what lies behind the Laughing Buddha Smile. At all times, remember, *"Dance with Fierce Hoopla!"*

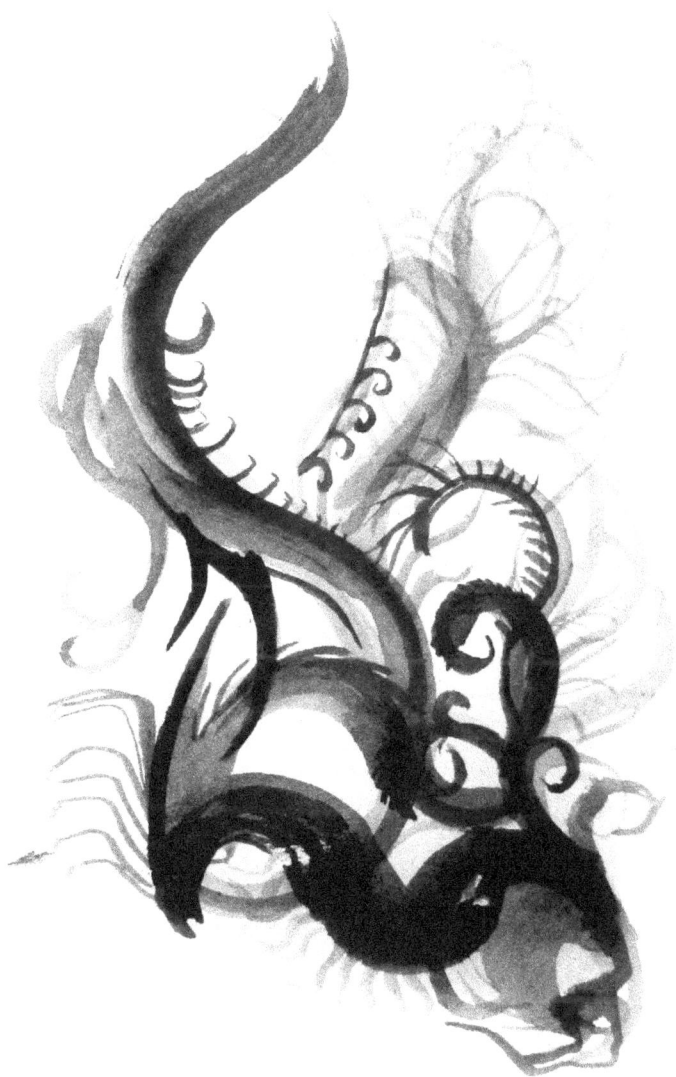

Part Four

Lightning and Thunder

20

Feel the Victory

American football players may be taught to "bite the football." This is a tackling technique taught from day one to the youngest of players. Unless a tackle is properly and safely executed, there is imminent danger of concussion/ mild traumatic brain injury or cervical vertebral fracture with resulting paralysis, and the technique of "biting the football" prevents the player from spearing his opponent with the helmet during a tackle. Players are instructed to keep their eyes on the football, or the player being tackled, at all times. The head should be up, but to the side of the player being tackled so that at the moment of contact it is possible to imagine biting the football. When a tackle is performed correctly, the tackle should be with the shoulder, not the face or helmet.

In order to take this training a step beyond the physical and into the world of chi, one must practice in a quiet setting. The intensity of hard physical tackles and competition is a distraction from chi nurturing and development. Once the practice of utilizing the chi has been mastered, it is then possible to incorporate this technique into the physical aspect of tackling. When one practices biting the football 'energetically,' an elevated amplitude of energy that will explode on contact is developed and tackles have more grace and "pop" than if reliance is on the physical body alone. Consciously exercising chi potential when tackling will also develop an Energetic Protective Shield around the head and neck.

Biting the football is a good introduction to the exploration of the practical use of teeth during mortal combat. The principle and training is the same: the goal is to drive and guide one's chi into the head, neck, face, mouth, teeth, jawbone, gums, and tongue. Once the chi that is being directed into these areas is sensed, or felt, begin pumping the chi like air into a tire to increase the pressure. (This is not the time or place to discuss the benefits of pumping chi into the teeth. Discussing the multiple benefits might plant suggestions, and it is better for the individual to experience and witness their own rewards.)

When I do this practice, I use imagination to take myself to the time of Ardi, and even beyond, to our unknown common ancestor. Simply biting a football in my present surroundings does not allow me to truly experience this technique. I visualize myself as primitive and naked, hair covering my body, hunting for food with my eyes wide open and all six senses fully alert! The hunted animal appears and suddenly I'm fighting—*life and limb, tooth and nail*—for my next meal. Muscles cut and flex, nerves tense, and I am "taking down" my prey with my teeth. Holding it in my vise-like jaw, I then drag it home to my family where my neck muscles fire one last time, slamming it down near the cooking fire. I experience a sense of strength and pride at the conclusion of another successful hunt.

This practice appears to be very physical, and the 'energetics' involved may not be initially perceptible. Before you can use your chi with purpose, you must first be able to **feel it.** When the mind and body are joined in a task, the feelings involved become imprinted onto the mind. Frequent repetition of the physical act will lead to very tangible mental sensations. After putting in some time with hard physical body motion, it becomes easy to see how soft mental imagination and visualization includes the solid, physical "chi feeling." Ultimately, using the mind alone, with no physical movement, will result in "feeling" the chi. Remember, it is best to practice alone in a quiet setting in order to focus on the imagination. Once the feeling becomes natural and spontaneous, add it into your game.

The simplest way to learn energy work is by one-on-one training with a teacher. Learning such techniques from a book alone is possible, but working with an experienced teacher makes for a more rapid and well-rounded learning experience. Experiencing chi transmission and reception is easier when an actual teacher is present—and the student is ready. For beginners attempting to get a feel for chi, I recommend the following schools/systems:

Taichi Tao Center *www.taichitaocenter.com*
Intended Evolution Fitness 150 *www.ifit150.com*

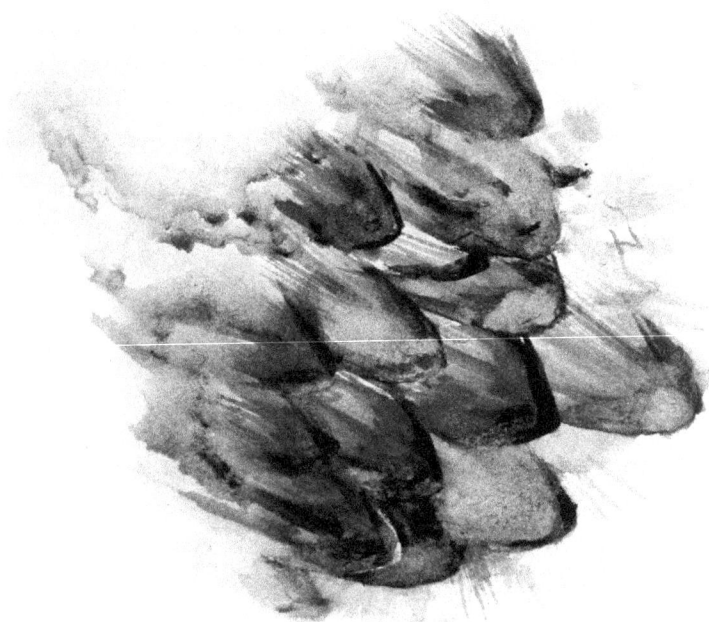

21

Relaxation with Determination

If you are serious about your martial arts, consider focusing some of your energy on the teeth and tongue. When teeth and tongue are incorporated into training, the wisdom behind the lips of The Laughing Buddha will become apparent. But The Laughing Buddha does not share his secrets with any who fail to follow these five rules:

> **Relax Completely**
> **Maintain Teeth Touching Lightly/Teeth Apart**
> **Touch Tip of Tongue to Palate**
> **Observe Posture**
> **Breathe with Diaphragm**

1. Relax Completely

How can one relax completely unless one also understands what it is to be completely tense? This is the way of energy—tense, relax, tense, relax, tense, relax. Chronic tension results in pain, disease, and death, but excessive relaxation leads to lethargy, depression, disease, and death. The secret to health, strength, vitality, and longevity is to lead a life of balance within varying degrees of tension and relaxation. During Teeth in Mortal Combat training, one utilizes tension and relaxation of the entire body, with special focus on the head and neck. Use the Predator-X jaw and Hex-Diamond White teeth to take down the prey, pick it up, and drop it at the cook's fire—and then relax. Attack and release. Tense and relax.

The first rule, to relax completely, may seem simple but there are many ways to relax, some more appropriate than others. It might be more accurate to use the term "relax correctly" rather than "relax completely." Learning to relax correctly can require much experimentation by the student and personal attention by an instructor. And one essential prerequisite of learning this skill is putting in a hard day's work.

For years I avoided stressful mental activities, strenuous exercise, and hard physical labor in order to grant myself as much time as possible to attempt to "relax completely." This was certainly another "mistake of inches" that led to my ending miles off course. What I have discovered, as the culmination of twenty-five years of trying to learn how to relax, is that the easiest and quickest way is to first work hard from dawn 'til dusk. At the end of the workday, when you are home and beginning to unwind, spend some time practicing and examining relaxation techniques. This will allow you to have a better understanding of what if feels like to relax and, more importantly, what it *means* to relax. Once you become accomplished at this, and add meditation to the mix, you can then apply the lessons learned into your hard working day—and I mean HARD work! Do not make the mistake of thinking that it is not possible to simultaneously work hard and relax. Work your fingers to the bone. Accomplish something with your life and be of service to the world.

I believe hard work in service will open your heart to the gift of deep relaxation. Remember, your work can become your meditation. Relaxation is a positive side effect of doing work and meditation correctly.

2. Teeth Apart

My tai chi teacher used to say, "The teeth should be lightly touching *and* not touching." Sometimes there was a slight variation: "The teeth should lightly touch *without* touching." I had no idea what he meant and I was paying him well to share his secrets with me. I did notice that he used the word "lightly" in both instructions. There must be some importance to touching *LIGHTLY*. To this day I do not know exactly what he meant. (If anyone can shed light on this for me, I would appreciate an email…)

I can, however, tell you what happens scientifically when one either clenches hard or "lightly" taps the teeth. Scientifically, we know that conscious *light* "tapping" of the teeth is a positive and healthy exercise that stimulates blood circulation in the root and surrounding bone. This helps eliminate the build up of toxins and improves the transport of nutrients to the teeth. Over time, lightly tapping the teeth during conscious exercise leads to greater bone mass and mineral density. Toxins are eliminated, nutrition improved, and overall regeneration and preservation of tissue is enhanced to extend the lifespan of the teeth.

Subconscious *hard* "clenching" over a long period of time leads to an opposite unhealthy result and can contribute to a shortened lifespan for the teeth. Clenching during martial arts training, if not done with caution and understanding, can become a serious tooth and health issue. The Temporal Mandibular Joint (TMJ) is a sensitive area consisting of nerves, arteries, and veins. When the masseter muscle clenches, the mandibular condyle compresses the TMJ joint bi-laminar area against the temporal fossa. Tetanic, tonic, or continuous muscle contraction with spasm of the masseter muscle eventually leads to an outstripping of the blood supply, lactic acid build-up, and fatigue of the muscles that close the jaw. Chronic and subconscious clenching may also harm the vital tissues in the TMJ joint as well as lead to soreness in the masseter and temporalis muscle. Clenching, without appropriate rest and recovery, may lead to pain and inflammation in the masseter and TMJ, and adjoining head, neck, and facial areas. Subconscious chronic clenching, or bruxism, often results in chronic headaches, visual disturbances, ear ringing, arthritis, limited jaw mobility, and loss of teeth.

Bruxism is the leading cause of occlusal trauma. It can result in abnormal tooth occlusal surface wear patterns, abfractions, and is extremely taxing on the tooth surface usually resulting in micro-fractures of the enamel surface. Over time the accumulation of micro-fractures may weaken the tooth enamel to the point of causing major cracks and chips. Often times in the mature adult, there is a non-restorable partial or complete splitting of the root structure resulting in loss of the tooth. This serious consequence is more common if the tooth has been hollowed out by previous decay or dental drilling. Chronic bruxism—clenching and grinding of teeth—is a significant factor in bone resorption, gum recession, and tooth loss.

Misaligned teeth interfere with the natural muscular movements of teeth sharpening. The long term effects could lead to teeth, jaw, head, neck, and shoulder pain. Ask your dentist to evaluate the smoothness of your bite and if there are any occlusive interferences. Consider any occlussal corrections your dentist might suggest, including orthodontics.

The stress of career, work, and relationships are contrib-uting factors to subconscious Bruxism. It is always best to address the problem of Bruxism before painful symptoms surface. Neutralize mental stress and bring balance into your life. Understand the Thegotic Theory of psychosocial suppression and find help in resolving the repression of the natural instinct to sharpen teeth.

Healthy muscles and bones in the jaw are essential. Mandibular Alveolar Bone Mass (MABM) measures inter-dental bone thickness. Skeletal Bone Mineral Density (BMD) refers to the amount of minerals in the bone such as calcium, magnesium, fluoride, and phosphorous. Greater bone mass and density makes for bone that is stronger and more resistant to fracture. The greater the MABM and BMD, the stronger and more resistant the bone is to stress fracture. Those among us who are desirous of a Predator-X steel jaw should attempt to increase both MABM and BMD with appropriate exercise and nutrition.

And studies have shown that masseter thickness and the number of occluding mandibular teeth were significant determinants of BMD. Masseter thickness occurs when the muscle is exercised and is a natural byproduct of eating hard and chewy foods, but it can also be due to the destructive subconscious habit of grinding and clenching. People with masseter thickness to the extent that it gives the appearance of a "square jaw" might want to examine if it is caused by pathological chronic bruxism or due to eating healthy, hard foods. Martial artists require a strong masseter with thick MABM and hard BMD in order to prevent jaw fracture during combat. Masseter thickness, MABM, and BMD may be increased by either safe teeth tapping or dangerous bruxing.

One way to positively affect the muscles, ligaments, and lymph around the face, jaw, and teeth is "tongue rolling." Tongue rolling stimulates salivary function, which is important for the exchange of minerals and waste between the enamel, dentin, and pulp tissue. It also energetically moves the chi within and around the teeth to increase vital function. This is a common chi kung technique, known to all knowledgeable instructors.

An important component of teeth, and one that is essential to dental health, is enamel. Human enamel is brittle: like glass, it cracks easily, but unlike glass, enamel is able to contain cracks and remain intact for the course of a lifetime. The major reason why teeth do not fracture and break apart is due to the presence of 'tufts'—small, crack-like defects found deep in the tooth at the dentin-enamel junction. These tufted cracks prevent major tooth chips and fractures due to trauma and biting by evenly distributing and absorbing the traumatic force.

Enamel also has a "basket weave" micro structure which protects against crack growth. Teeth possess a self-healing process wherein organic material fills cracks extending from the tufts. This type of infilling bonds opposing crack walls and increases the amount of force needed to break the tooth. Safe teeth tapping utilizes this unique self-healing aspect to rebuild and strengthen teeth. Martial artists make use of this natural crack-healing ability to rebuild and strengthen the body so that they can break baseball bats with their shinbones, or bricks with their hands and heads. Similar results may be obtained through teeth tapping, and a healthy tooth should easily crack walnuts and other hard-shelled foods. If you want to change your glass jaw into one of steel, it helps to understand these modern scientific principles while you incorporate ancient chi kung training techniques. Strong healthy teeth are your main source of resistance training for increasing masseter strength, bone mass, and bone density.

Tapping the teeth and conscious clenching, when practiced correctly, are the beginning techniques of Teeth in Mortal Combat training. Teeth tapping vibrates the hard yet supple tooth structure and associated fluids setting up shock waves that help push the toxic waste out. Teeth tapping also strengthens the tooth structure against the impact of daily biting, chewing, and grinding. Conscious light "tapping" of your teeth improves chi energy and blood circulation through the roots, gums, and bone. Over time, lightly tapping the teeth during exercise leads to greater bone mass and mineral density. Toxins are eliminated, nutrition improved, and overall regeneration and preservation of body tissue is enhanced to extend the lifespan of the teeth. As one progresses, the intensity of tapping and clenching naturally builds, so in order to safely increase masseter thickness and strength, as well as MABM and BMD, healthy molar and premolar teeth are of vital importance.

You may be wondering why most of this section has been devoted to teeth touching even though its title is "Teeth Apart." There is a good reason for this seeming anomaly: I want to emphasize the physical dangers of both conscious and subconscious teeth touching when practiced without guidance. Many people make the mistake of initially biting or tapping with too much force, or acquiring the bad habit of bruxism. Teeth touching is serious business and mistakes can result in permanent damage to your teeth, bone, and jaw.

Training *teeth apart,* however, is very safe and innocuous. The easiest way to train "teeth apart" is to take a few seconds and step away from what you are doing and then "yawn, smile, swallow your saliva, relax." If your mouth is dry, take a sip of water or put something sweet or sour into your mouth. One goji berry or a small piece of lemon peel is all it takes to activate the salivary glands.

There are times throughout the day when your teeth naturally touch or do not touch. For example, when you swallow it is normal for the teeth to lightly touch, but when you yawn, the teeth do not touch. Relax and know that most of the day you are in the groove. See this natural reflex every time you drink a beverage or swallow your saliva. This is the physical level to explain the instruction, "the teeth should be lightly touching and not touching."

If you find it difficult to relax and keep your teeth apart, then focus more on the tongue. Concentrating on the tongue can signal the salivary glands to secrete more saliva—a Yin process—which may then be swallowed so its healing chi may be absorbed by lower dan-tien, signalling the nervous system to restore peace and calm. Pent up repressive emotions melt and the teeth and jaws relax. As a result, the teeth will tend to stay apart, coming together with only the minimum necessary force indicated for proper function... Life is beautiful!

Masters give such instruction as focusing on the tongue to help the student free the mind from the world of attached thoughts. This is called "taming the wild horse." Placing the focus of the mind on an immediate puzzle does not allow for thoughts of the past or future. It anchors one in the present moment, where the only reality exists.

Conscious awareness of "teeth apart" is necessary for the brain to make the appropriate changes, and in order to be aware of "teeth apart," it helps to first have them touch lightly. Joining a meditation class can be very helpful. You know the old saying, "Success comes with numbers."

Remember the mantra:

Lips Together, Teeth Apart
Relax, Smile and Open Your Heart!

3. Tongue on Palate

Most meditations require lightly placing the tip of the tongue on the upper palate. There are a number of reasons for this: the tongue is a very energy-sensitive muscle and serves as a conduit for language, cognitive thought, and emotional experiences such as suckling, tasting, and sexual pleasure. Activate the mind and the tongue prepares itself to express the thoughts. As previously mentioned, the tongue, heart, and mind are energetically associated, and the tongue also is used to form a bridge connecting the Conception and Governing vessels. But unless the tongue has a purpose during active meditation, it can prove to be a distraction. Assigning this simple task to the tongue allows the mind to remain more focused and makes it easier to find the quiet space within.

A more medical reason to press the tongue on the roof of the mouth is related to sinus problems. It is commonly believed that pressing hard on the upper palate with the thumb of one hand, and then using the palm of the other hand to press firmly on the spot between the eyes, can 'rock' the sinus. Alternating the pressure between the two spots for twenty seconds creates a rocking vibration that will cause some movement of the nasal and vomer (a facial bone just atop the palate) bones to open the sinus and allow congestion to drain. I believe that just pressing the tongue against the roof of the mouth will create a similar effect, allowing the air and energy to circulate more freely through the nose and sinus. A free flow of breath and energy are helpful during both quiet meditation and physical exercise.

The upper palate is a fairly large space and there are various locations, depending on one's purpose, where the tongue tip may be placed. A good starting point is the "cluck" position: make a "clucking" sound and see where the tongue touches the palate in order to produce that sound. (For dental professionals reading this, if the "cluck" feels too "ducky," then perform a zygomatic smile, slide into centric relation, lightly touch the teeth together, and bring the tip of the tongue up to touch the palate somewhere between the central and posterior region. You will have no trouble finding the "sweet" spot as it feels like sipping sweet nectar.) When the tongue is pressed against the roof of the mouth or above the front teeth of the upper palate, the chi is activated and a strong connection between the mind and tongue is established. By holding the tongue in a stable position against the palate, the activated chi can be harnessed and directed for purposes other than speaking.

When the tongue is relaxed and allowed to rest in the center of the mouth without touching the palate, the chi is also activated, but with a different purpose. Thoughts immediately slow down while potential energy accumulates in various storage chambers. This is the difference between active and passive meditation. In both cases, either with the tongue relaxed and not touching the palate, or with the tongue touching the palate, the activity of the mind calms down. In active meditation the quieted mind is prepped, much like drawing an arrow back in a bow, harnessing the energy in preparation to shoot. In passive meditation, the still mind watches the universe move within and without; there is no intention to shoot, but the potential exists and it can change at any moment.

Try it. Close your eyes and relax your tongue and you will notice how quickly your mind softens and relaxes and the chi accumulates. This helps you in your passive meditation. If you are practicing specific active meditations, press the tongue on the roof of the mouth and sense how your energy activates and strengthens. When your tongue touches the upper palate, the elixirs in saliva flow and, when swallowed, drain into and fill lower dan-tien. Use the mind to stoke the fire in the dan-tien in order to purify and transmute the elixir.

The tongue position is reflexively controlled by jaw position (the jaw-tongue reflex). During combat, one needs to protect the jaw by retruding it, or moving and holding it in the most rearward position. This is possible because of the multi-dimensional nature of the TMJ which functions to hold and move the jaw into its many versatile positions. When the mandible is retruded, the tongue reflexively moves into the best position for bridging the upward and downward flowing energy pathways within the oral cavity. In dentistry, this retruded position is called "centric relation."

Swallowing also reflexively moves the tongue into the ideal place for meditation. Many meditations call for one to 'swallow' imaginary objects such as the sun, moon, flames, watery elixirs, pearls, etc. Swallowing helps one to become more familiar with the tongue's energy and how it engages with the other energies flowing in and around the oral cavity. It is valuable to watch and feel how the different parts of the oral cavity interact while these meditations are performed.

There are many different optimal positions for the tongue to occupy depending on the specific practice. But when involved in mortal combat, the last thing a combatant needs to worry about is tongue placement. One's instinct should take care of this detail, allowing one to focus entirely on survival and victory. During combat, the tongue should instinctively and subconsciously be controlled so as to prevent accidental self-biting. A blow to the face can force the mandible upward with great momentum, causing a severe bite to the tongue. Placing the tongue upward against the center of the palate, or curling it down behind the lower front teeth, will prevent such a traumatic injury. This is another reason to practice pressing it against the roof of the mouth. If this instinct is repressed, repetitious practice is necessary to reawaken this technique.

When preparing for combat, it is important to marshal all of the various instinctive survival energies. Like a complex energy grid at times of intense overload, certain energy pathways are required to shut down in order to direct the maximum amount of energy to the meridians and organs used for self-preservation; having active digestive energy during a fight for life is counterproductive. (During training it is necessary to be conscious of the amount of chi and pressure in the various meridians in order to prevent damage—in the form of an 'energetic aneurysm'—from occurring. Working one-on-one with a qualified instructor is vital to adequately mastering this aspect of chi management.)

When training for mortal combat, the tendency is to bite and clench the teeth to extremes, which can lead to damaging the teeth. One method to solve this problem is to rely on the Yin energy of the tongue to contain the exuberant Yang energy of the teeth. During peak periods of physical practice, press the tongue hard against the roof of the mouth. When the tongue is pressed into the upper palate with sufficient strength, the teeth are unable to clench with maximum force. The pressure with the tongue will vary depending on the practice, and with trial and error it is possible to achieve the proper and comfortable balance between tongue pressure and teeth biting force. Another trick to keep the teeth from clenching too hard is to bring the teeth lightly together and then inhale through the mouth and front teeth as if sucking the air into the mouth through the spaces between the teeth. It should create a "hissing" sound when the tongue is properly placed.

The only appropriate time to have the teeth biting down with maximum force is when there is something between the jaws, such as a hunted animal, or an opponent's body part. During training, when there is nothing between the teeth and tooth-to-tooth contact is being made, make certain to press the tongue against the palate with enough pressure to prevent compressive bite force injury to the teeth. *Never, for any reason or at any time, clench to the limit during visualization and imagination exercises.* This could easily cause dental-facial trauma such as cracked teeth, broken fillings and crowns, TMJ injury, and lockjaw.

I believe that even though the tongue channels energy more efficiently while in contact with the roof of the mouth, there may be more distraction in telling a novice to do so than there is benefit to be gained. At the very beginning of your practice, it is acceptable to just let the tongue relax and have it rest behind the top two front teeth. As you proceed, integrate the more complicated techniques in a logical, comfortable progression in order to avoid injury.

4. Posture

Development of one's posture depends upon genetics, the birth experience as one enters the world, and the effects of emotions on the body as we grow and mature. Many books addressing perfect posture have been written, but reading is not enough: one must first be aware of posture and then consciously work to correct it. My personal experiences with working on posture may be of some help.

I tried for twenty-five years to consciously improve my posture by tucking in the tailbone, pulling up the perineum, imagining a string attached to and pulling up the crown point at the top of my skull, balancing books on the top of the head, etc. These methods were effective—up to a point—but nothing worked as well as simple sprinting and walking on my toes. I became more aware of my posture after walking on the balls and toes of my feet for two or three miles at a time. My awareness improved further by sprinting short distances of about fifty yards on the balls of my feet. I did both of the above at least twice a week for several months. Try it and observe your results.

It is interesting to note that babies innately know to begin ambulation with the "toddler walk" and to run on the balls of their feet. As they mature, they start to imitate their parents and begin walking heel-to-toe. Which is correct or preferable: heel-to-toe or toe-to-heel? I am not qualified to answer that question, but I do believe there is benefit in watching babies use what the gurus call "no mind." I vary my walking style in order to hone my awareness.

Try walking and sprinting on the balls of your feet. It works wonders to improve posture!

5. Breathe with Diaphragm

Full breathing with the diaphragm is the fundamentally most important exercise for one to perform in order to achieve progress in all areas of chi development. Many various types of breathing exercises that have originated in China and India are now being taught and practiced in the West. In order to gain valuable exposure to as many of these as possible, it is necessary to work with a teacher who has a strong background in chi kung and/or pranayama breathing techniques. At the time of this writing, David Blaine holds the world record for holding his breath and a number of his excellent breathing exercises may be found online.

I strongly suggest that you find a teacher who will safely guide you through the finer points of breathing exercises. One bit of advice I can contribute is to place your hand on your stomach and feel the abdomen expand outward with the inhale and contract inward with the exhale. In some practices, the desired effect is the opposite—the stomach expands outward on the exhale and contracts inward with the inhale.

I would like to share with you an exercise that will enhance your awareness of breath and chi and simultaneously benefit the diaphragm, teeth and nervous system:

1. Purchase a pair of Vibram Five Finger, FeelMax Niesa, mocassin, or any other similar style of barefoot running or walking shoe. This type of shoe is the best that I have found to help me connect with the energy of the earth while still protecting the soles of my feet.

2. Stand comfortably and clasp the fingers of your hands together and rest them on top of the head.

3. Keep the teeth apart and lightly press the tip of the tongue onto the roof of the mouth.

4. Breathe through the nose. If you are unable to breathe smoothly through the nose, breathe through the mouth.

5. Tense the perineum slightly—and definitely avoid clenching tightly—so you can locate it and feel the energy move up the spine.

6. Relax the entire body—and pay special attention to relaxing the abdomen—bend the knees slightly, and start walking very slowly backwards.

7. Coordinate your breaths with each step. Inhale while taking one step backward, exhale on the next step backward. Repeat in a rhythmic pattern. (As you become comfortable with this technique, you can play with different rhythms of breathing and stepping.)

8. Continue in this manner until you have your balance and are relatively relaxed.

9. Relax the abdomen, allow the teeth to touch lightly, and step backward slowly. With each step, inhale the

breath in stages, a little at a time: breathe first into the perineum, then the lower abdomen, and continue to inhale in increments until the breath fills the upper abdomen, the solar plexus, middle chest area, and continue this process until the upper chest and shoulders are completely filled with air. At this point the entire torso, from perineum to shoulders, is completely filled with air.

10. With the next step *explode* all of the air out through the nose or mouth in this manner: pull up on the perineum, contract the abdomen inward toward the spine, compress the rib cage, pull the shoulders down, and interlock the fingers strongly down onto the head. Most importantly, the abdomen should fire backwards like a piston, striking against the front of the spine.

11. Repeat this pattern until you tire of it and then turn around, relax, and start walking forward. Continue breathing and exploding in a more relaxed manner and with a reduced measure of horsepower. Imagine that when you begin the exercise you are in neutral, release the clutch and explode into first gear, then second, third, and fourth gear. When you tire, turn around and start walking forward and shift into fifth gear, coasting comfortably while you regain your composure and energy. The piston does not have to slap the spine while you are in fifth gear. When you feel re-energized, turn around and start walking backward again and repeat the steps.

12. You should spend most of your time enjoying the recovery stage in fifth gear, coasting comfortably while taking in the fresh air and enjoying nature. When you feel the time is right for another explosion, turn around and

begin walking backward, drop down into neutral and explode with all of your accessible horsepower into first gear, second, and so on until turning around and walking forward again in 5th gear.

Fifth gear is most enjoyable and it is very important that you spend most of your time there. Figure 5–10% of the time for first gear, 10–20% for second, third, and fourth combined, and 70–80% for fifth gear. Use this opportunity to become more in touch with your chi: when you tire, do not use your will power and force yourself to drop down and explode again into first gear. Wait until your chi "tells" you that recovery is complete, the tank is topped off, and the engine and driver are ready. Recognize and pay attention to your chi communicating with you. The mind and will are very powerful and may easily convince you to start too soon, before the chi is ready. ***Listen to your chi in order to gain the most benefit.***

Forward walking is where the barefoot running shoe reveals its significant advantage over conventional walking, jogging, or running shoes. As you step forward, hit the heel **HARD** on the ground. The impact will transfer earth energy through the thin rubber sole and send a vibration upward through the skeletal bones from the heel to the leg, up through the spine to the neck and skull, finally connecting with the mandible by way of the TMJ. The vibration ends with the teeth gently clashing against each other and the teeth will begin to vibrate in rhythm with the steps. This creates a cool experience that is very healthy and invigorating for the whole body, including the brain.

You will discover remarkable benefits for the teeth. When you feel the teeth vibrating, know that your brain cells are also are being affected in a positive way by the vibrational frequency. Your entire central nervous system begins to rewire itself into a higher level of potential energy conduction.

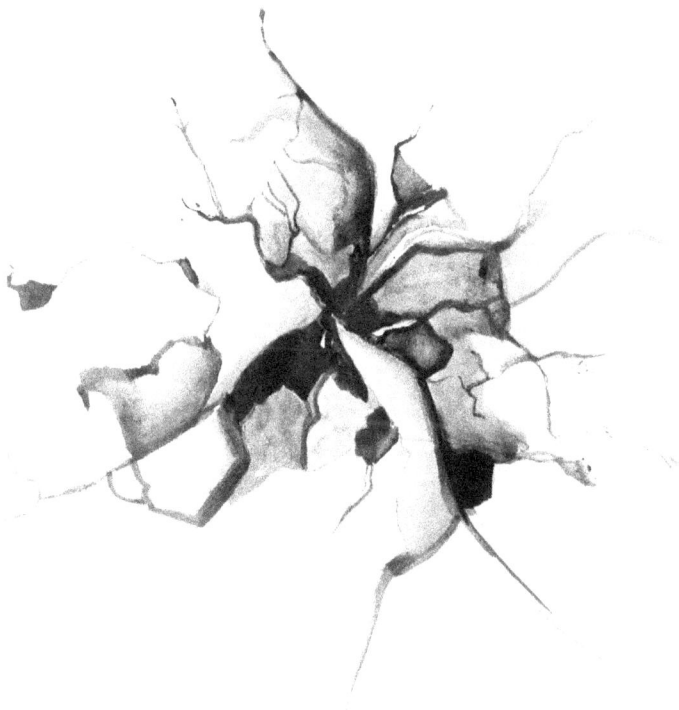

22

Athletic Mouth Guards and Helmets

The conventional wisdom has it that athletic mouth guards are important for safety and protection of the mouth and teeth, and that mouth guards are an essential piece of protective gear for athletes who play contact sports. Accordingly, an athletic mouth guard not only protects the teeth, but the soft tissue around the mouth area that may be damaged by the teeth. I agree, in a limited way, with these statements.

Helmets are likewise viewed as essential prophylaxis for preventing head injuries. An estimated 1.6 to 3.8 million recreation-related concussions are sustained annually in the United States, many of them on football fields. When children and teens suffer a concussion, they must be strictly monitored and their activities restricted. They should never under any circumstances return to the field of play, and no cognitive activities such as reading and studying for school, text messaging, video games or television are allowed until they have fully recovered.

The problem today is that sports-related concussions in children and athletes often go unrecognized and often do not receive proper respect for their potential seriousness. A concussion is actually—mild traumatic brain injury. A recent study found that if a child is given a diagnosis of concussion, parents treat it more lightly than if it is spoken more correctly as "mild traumatic brain injury." The change in language by medical doctors could help protect the child from returning to school sooner than recommended. One study of U.S. college athletes who had concussions indicated suppressed brain function more than three years later.

Newly redesigned helmets show promise to further protect the skull from splitting, although they still cannot prevent an athlete's brain from rattling around inside the skull like a scrambled yolk inside an eggshell. But more and more studies are revealing that mouth guards, helmets, etc. are NOT protecting contact sport athletes from long-term negative health consequences. *They are only providing a false sense of security.*

American football is one of the most dangerous sports on the planet because of the false sense of safety that mouth guards and helmets generate. Repetitive hits to the body, even with protective body armor, usually impart a concussive force to the skeletal structure, spinal cord, and brain. An athlete, after just one season, can end up with permanent physical and mental damage that will go unnoticed until later in life. It is little wonder that professional football players have recently begun to donate their brains to science so that the long-term effects of multiple concussions may be studied.

Australian Rules Football has a no-helmet rule, yet their players have twenty-five percent fewer head injuries than helmeted American players. This one statistic alone should raise a red flag about the consequences of wearing a helmet. The false sense of security a helmet provides drives athletes to 'spear' opponents with their heads. Spearing is very dangerous to all involved, and head injuries, immediate and delayed, almost always result. In my opinion, helmets should be banned from American football. And until that comes to pass, spearing with the helmet should be disciplined by banning the offending player from the sport for life.

Head injuries are also much more likely to occur when a fatigued or injured player enters the game, and in the world of multi-million dollar pro contracts, little is done to prevent this from happening. Head injuries, even if asymptomatic at game time, may remain passive in nature until they erupt like a boil years later. Symptoms of brain concussion injuries, often dormant when young, begin to show themselves in many athletes by the time they reach their early thirties.

If athletes must wear mouth guards to protect their teeth, then they are playing with fear, fatigue, or injury. If one is fearless and fresh, one's reflexes will be fully active and one's chi should protect against serious injuries. A player with fresh, active chi does not need a mouth guard or a helmet. I believe there would be fewer head and teeth injuries if players were trained to use their chi to protect themselves from injury. Of course, this scenario is dependent upon the assumption that athletes are aware of their chi and paying attention to its subtle messages as to whether it is fatigued or unable to fully protect them. Coaches are certainly also responsible for keeping fatigued and injured players out of the game. Common sense combined with heightened chi awareness is the solution to many serious athletic injuries.

In my opinion, American football—as it is played with helmet, body padding, and mouth guard—comes very close to fitting the description of mortal combat because of the possible long-term negative effects on the brain. **I support mortal combat in only two instances: one is in life and**

death situations, and the other is in training for survival. *Teeth in Mortal Combat* prepares a warrior for those specific scenarios; it is not to be used for sport and play. I do not believe in or support spectator sports involving anything close to mortal combat for amusement. Survival for one's life is VERY serious business, not entertainment to be had with beer and chips on the side.

Returning to the topic of mouth guards, I would like to highlight some facts about their usage and how they ultimately interfere with the development of chi in the teeth, jaws, and tongue. The TMJ is the most active joint in the body, as it is used for breathing, chewing, swallowing, and speaking. Keeping the joint healthy and free of injury should be of primary importance to martial artists, but wearing a mouth guard does not help in this regard. On the contrary, it actually interferes with the body's natural innate patterns of self-preservation.

First, it is important to note that when we bite down, we are not literally biting *down.* The top teeth do not bite downward, rather it is the bottom teeth and jaw that are biting upward. Upward biting plays an important role in the development and utilization of chi in the mouth because it requires one to draw upon the upward flowing energy of the conception vessel. The downward flowing energy of the governing vessel stabilizes the head and keeps the upper teeth positioned for contact with the lower. When the two energies meet, there is a dynamic whirlpool of potential energy in the head, neck, and mouth area.

(So how did the phrase "bite down" originate? We do know that the idiom "bite the dust" means to fall down dead. My guess is that many thousands of years ago, long before the advent of bows or firearms, combatants who bit the dust did so because their opponent forcefully smashed them down to the ground, similar to the meaning of the phrase "take down" used in wrestling. The phrase "bite down" was eventually modernized and applied to any biting of the jaw and teeth.)

I believe there is the memory of our original ancient ancestor stored in the energetic blueprint of our jaw, and that we can tap into it during mortal combat. And I am quite certain that this ancestor possessed a biting mechanism that was ripe with chi potential and likewise depended on the jaw and teeth for self-defense during mortal combat to a tremendous extent. In order to awaken this powerful function within ourselves, we can do some simple exercises and visualizations. The tongue, as mother to the teeth, plays a role in this awakening process by helping to open up the entire system, including the psyche, to respond to commands. It releases inner strength and abolishes fear.

When one wears a mouth guard, the teeth and lower jaw are splinted into a fixed position and the tongue is prevented from freely touching the teeth. One of the first rules in chi development is to allow the mind, body, and spirit to relax, be flexible, and move freely.

(Naturally, if one is injured or disabled and needs to wear some type of a cast, splint, or brace in order to heal an injury, there are methods available to access healing chi while one is bound by these medical necessities. An injured player, however, should never be allowed onto the playing field as this only puts the weakened player in harm's way and interferes with the healing process. A healthy, fully capable athlete should, on the other hand, never wear a cast, brace, or padding into the arena. If the brace or padding is being worn to avoid possible injury, then it might be time to examine the purpose of the game. Is the game designed to uplift the human spirit and condition? In what ways do the rules advance or hinder the emotional and spiritual growth of the player? What is the relationship between player and spectator? Does the spectator gain twisted pleasure in seeing pain and bloodshed on the field of play?)

One of the beautiful qualities of the tongue is that it communicates with the energy system of the entire body through its contact with the teeth, which have meridians of every organ system in the body running through them. Rubbing the tip of the tongue against all of the tooth surfaces is not only a way to clean the teeth, but it is the method through which the mother tongue connects with the whole body. Rubbing the teeth is also pleasurable to the tongue and strengthens and stimulates it. The salivary glands begin to secrete a higher volume of elixir into the mouth, lubricating the tongue and teeth for even greater pleasure. If you desire a happy, healthy tongue, stimulate it daily by rubbing it against your teeth. Mouth guards serve only to interfere with this natural pleasure.

The universal rule is that a chain is only as strong as its weakest link. This is why we must pay special attention to the jaw if our goal is to increase physical strength. For overall maximum physical output, every part of the body has to function at its optimum ability. In order to kick, punch, or block to maximum effect, the jaw must be freely held in its ideal functioning position so that no link is kinked. The chi must be unrestricted and flowing with full potential through every link in the chain. And in order for the chi to fully protect the teeth and jaw, the mandible must also be perfectly positioned. This position varies according to the posture of the whole body, whether leaning forward, backward, to the left, to the right, stooping, crouching or standing on one leg. The lower jaw position of greatest strength will vary, depending on the angle of the head on the cervical spine. Mouth guards in this situation will interfere with freedom of movement.

The strength of the masseter muscle is directly related to the position of the mandible within the space of the TMJ, and protrusive force directions gain the highest relative activation of the masseter. The posterior deep muscle region of the masseter seems to possess the most active fibers during clenching and biting. This means that one must move the lower jaw slightly forward to find the location of greatest available strength, or 'sweet spot', for the task at hand.

And essential to correct positioning of the jaw, the TMJ is one of the most complex joints in the body. All body parts move with some rotation and circular motion and the jaw is no different; it opens and closes with more than a simple hinged motion. When the jaw is searching for the sweet spot, it will maneuver on multiple axes in a manner that cannot be seen by the naked eye. When the teeth and mandible are locked into a mouth guard, there is no opportunity for the jaw to search for and vibrate into the sweet spot. Finding the sweet spot for maximum strength happens subconsciously, instinctively, reactively, and instantaneously, through constant adjustments to changes in posture and the angle of the head on the cervical spine. The mandible must be free to glide in all directions in order to chomp into the prize with maximum force. It also is a vital link that must remain unimpeded so that other parts of the body can deliver the maximum output of energy—an impossibility if one is saddled with a restrictive mouth guard. Although professional athletes wear mouth guards that are custom made by dentists, it is not possible for the dentist to locate or duplicate the floating sweet spot in an appliance.

Do not rely on helmets, padding, and mouth guards to protect your body, as they only impart a false sense of security at best. They cannot teach your chi to *explode outward.* If you choose to nurture your inner self and strengthen your physical body through athletic endeavors, then participate in sports that give you the freedom to achieve those ends. Find a sport that enables you to access and learn from your chi while simultaneously developing and protecting it. Avoid sports that place your chi in harm's way. Use your chi wisely.

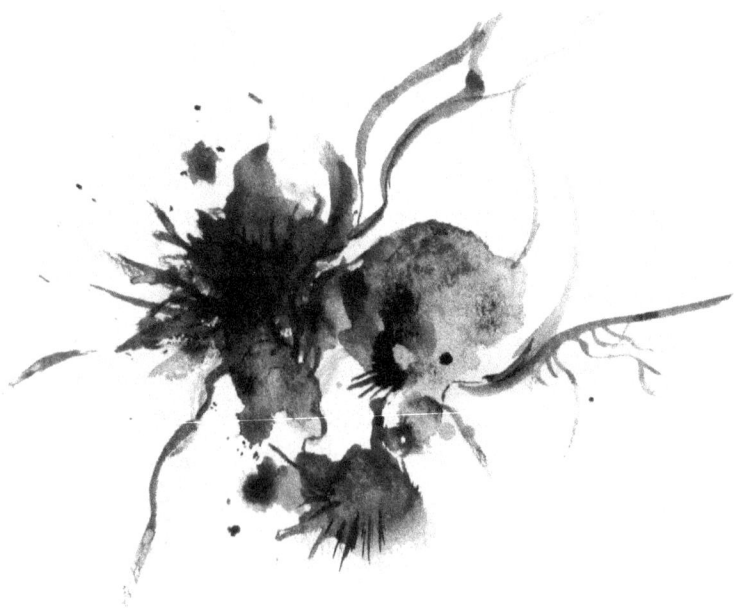

23

Wine and Dreams

Professor Cheng Man-ch'ing was considered, by many, to be the "Mater of Five Excellencies," including Chinese medicine, tai chi chuan, calligraphy, painting, and poetry. In the United States he was most popular for his martial arts ability of unleashing power through his thumbs. When asked how he learned the ability to transfer chi power through an opponent, he would say that *he had a dream in which his arms fell off.* In my humble opinion, dreams are often used to explain away mysterious secrets that a person does not want to share with you. For example, where did I glean the information that has become *Teeth in Mortal Combat?* Well, most of it presented in dreams...

I have listened to a number of eyewitness accounts from American and Chinese martial artists who have studied in China. According to them, many of the chi masters in China drink alcohol as if it were water, smoke tobacco like chimneys, and use narcotics such as opium. This is not surprising considering the fact that, based on evidence uncovered at archaeological sites, opium appears to be a substance of long-standing ritual significance. Anthropologists have speculated that ancient priests may have used the drug as a proof of healing power. Wine, hemp and hallucinogenics are other intoxicants used by spiritual seekers to access higher planes of knowledge. When someone tells me that they acquired information in a dream, I am always interested in learning about the circumstances around the dream-state.

I doubt very much that this occurs during the typical REM dream-state experienced by most people every night.

I want to share an epiphany with you, one not associated with a dream-state: when I imagined that my arms had fallen off and I began to visualize fighting a wild animal with my teeth, *a whole new world of possibilities opened up for me.* After I visualized fighting with my teeth and began to incorporate an intense zygomatic smile into my practice, the power of the Laughing Buddha filled my head, neck, oral cavity, teeth, and jaws. My top and bottom halves connected with my bottom, right side separated from left side, front became clear against back.

You, too, can have a similar experience: Visualize your arms shackled behind your back and fight with your teeth. Hiss like the snake, prowl like the tiger, growl with the lion. Use your teeth to take down, choke, pull, push, pin against a tree, throw into the river. Take the yoke between your teeth and pull the plow freely. Work the field. Lift the earth, swing the moon, fish the stars. Release an invisible net of chi from your mouth, hook and sinker baited with instinct.

This is what I call a "Dance with Fierce Hoopla!"

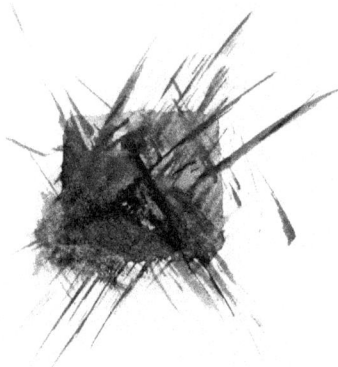

24

Basic Training Instruction

Training teeth and jaws involves certain risks and I strongly caution everyone interested in attempting to use the exercises portrayed on my website, *www.Tooth-Fight.com,* to first undergo complete and thorough dental and medical examinations. *This chapter contains the only written instructions for the exercise training videos on my website. Watching the videos in combination with reading this chapter should answer all of your questions on how to practice.* **Attempting to study and practice the exercises shown on the videos without reading this book—or vice versa—may be harmful to your health.**

Fresh air is an essential ingredient to a healthy training session. If practicing inside, crack open a window or door. It is preferable to train barefoot or wear an ultra-thin soled shoe like a moccasin or barefoot running shoe. Avoid urinating after training for at least 20 minutes to help prevent dissipating any chi accumulated during the session.

It is recommended to use silk fabric for this training. Silk is a natural protein fiber very similar to human hair and our bodies respond far better to silk than they do to synthetic products. Natural amino acids in the silk fiber are very similar to human hair. It is naturally hypoallergenic and is mold and mildew resistant due to its ability to wick away moisture. Because of its smooth surface, its frictional coefficient is only 7.4%, which is the lowest among all fibers. It is relatively resistant to aging. It is best to buy silk colored with natural dyes and dyestuffs made from plants, minerals, and insects. The silk should be about three feet wide and the length of your body. Fold the silk onto itself three times in order to get a comfortable fit.

Lesson One: Warm-up

1a) Be certain as many teeth as possible are biting into the silk. Hold the silk with your hands below your head. As you inhale slowly, pull the silk upward and extend the neck comfortably as far back as possible. Hesitate a moment, then exhale slowly and completely as you pull the chin down toward your chest. Hesitate a moment then repeat several times.

1b) This time repeat the instructions in 1a) holding the silk in your hands above your head.

2a) Face straight ahead, keep both arms outstretched at your sides, and inhale completely. Exhale slowly as you pull the silk to the right as far as your neck will allow, then try turning a bit more to see behind you as you completely expel all the remaining air in your lungs. Hesitate a moment, then begin inhaling slowly while using your teeth to pull the silk back to the starting position. Hesitate a moment and then repeat again several times.

2b) Follow the same procedure turning the head to the opposite side.

Lesson Two: Squat and Rise

Be absolutely sure that you tie your silk securely to the doorknob and that the door is firmly closed, locked, or bolted and that it is impossible for the door to come open. Clear the area behind you so that if your bite grip, silk tie knot, door lock or jamb accidentally are compromised, there will be no injury should you fall backward.

Begin by standing close to the door and maintaining a fairly vertical body position while holding the silk with both hands. As you become stronger and more confident, increase the backward lean and release your grip on the silk. Eventually and **ideally, you want to keep your hands folded over your lower abdomen.**

Open your eyes wide and maintain a zygomatic smile. Inhale completely and then slowly exhale as you squat down as far as comfort allows. The motion should be teeth pulling the chin towards the chest. Expel all the air from your lungs, hesitate, and then slowly rise as you breathe into and try to expand your lower abdomen. When you approach your starting position, arch your spine and neck backward as the shoulders pull back and complete your inhale by expanding the chest wall in all directions as much as comfort allows. Hesitate a moment, then repeat squatting and rising several times.

Lesson Three: Completion—Sealing Chi

Stand with feet apart slightly wider than shoulder width. Imagine a heavy barbell resting at your feet and that a weighted object such as a heavy pillow is between your teeth. The teeth DO NOT clench! Breathe through your teeth and create a 'shi' sound.

Eyes are wide open with a zygomatic smile and knees are slightly bent. Inhale completely, then exhale and bend over to pick up the heavy barbell while holding the weighted pillow between your teeth. *The teeth ALWAYS lead the movement. In other words, the teeth lift the pillow just slightly before you pick up the barbell. Always keep your focus on the teeth.* Inhale and pull the barbell to your waist and fling the pillow up and behind your head. **Your spine and neck are arched back, shoulders are pulled back, and your chest is full of air.** Hold your breath as long as possible while you swallow any saliva in your mouth down into your lower dan-tien. (If your mouth is dry, try to force a swallow into your dan-tien or lower abdomen. It is normal to adjust your head and neck from the extended position in order to swallow.) While still firmly holding the barbell at your waist, exhale as you bend forward and use your teeth to whip the pillow from behind your head and slam it to the ground. The imaginary barbell always remains in your hands. Exhale completely and repeat the motion up and back, hold your breath, swallow, and slam the pillow down.

At the point where you cannot swallow anymore, continue with a couple more movements without the swallow.

Always end the exercise in the physical stance you started from: standing straight up with knees slightly bent, but with a final seal where you force a complete exhale by pulling the shoulders forward and down while simultaneously pulling up the hui-yin/perineum and contracting the lower abdomen.

AND REMEMBER: THE TEETH ALWAYS lead the movement. (Imagine a large whip stock between your teeth as you control the whip.)

When you tire, take a short break and then repeat a few more times until your chi tells you it is time to end. The best time to end is when you are beginning to feel slightly tired, but still energized, happy, and fulfilled. Focus on any good feelings you experience as you recover. Tell yourself, "Golly, this feels good." Enjoy the moment of increased vital energy.

25

Live Again—Totally FREE!

The martial arts are intended to be a tough, mean, no holds barred combat for survival. Sharp teeth and massive jaws, when developed for martial arts, are lethal weapons born of pure animal instinct. In my opinion, nothing displays more clearly the most fearsome wildness in man's nature than his usage of jaws and teeth for assault and self-defense.

Spectators at today's sporting events do not even flinch when one athlete combatant breaks an opponent's arm, jaw, wrist, or gouges an eye. However, if one athlete uses teeth to rip into the flesh, muscle or sinew of another, the media and fans are quick to brand the offender as a barbarian or, even worse, something sub-human. One has to ask why society bans the use of teeth in self-defense. The awareness and development of the basic instinct of biting for self-defense is stifled at an early age and propriety insists that the awesome and brutal capabilities of teeth and jaws are not even proper subjects for discussion in 'polite society'. What is behind this subjugation, oppression and control of natural instinct?

The taboo on biting is world-wide, and many colorful theories have been contrived to support the various reasons for universal complicity. The theory that I find most interesting—from a mechanical, physiological, biological, and energetic point of view—is revealed in the musings of *Reversing the Curse* by Jean-Claude Koven. According to Koven, the Anunnuki were an alien species that visited

Earth at the time when our solar system was beginning to form. They needed to mine our gold, ship it back to their mother planet and, through an elaborate process, disperse it into their atmosphere in order to restore habitable oxygen levels. The mine laborers rebelled at some point and the Anunnuki leaders decided to replace them with one of Earth's own native species, homo erectus. This solution proved unsatisfactory so the Anunnuki performed genetic engineering to splice genes from our own homo erectus with their native genes. The result was a hybrid species, homo sapiens, which proved perfect for mining.

But there were further problems with interbreeding and uncontrolled population growth. War broke out and the Anunnuki decided on a plan to tame the uncontrollable new species they created in order to allow peace to prevail. They deliberately engineered a genetic code into homo sapiens that would transform their new pool of mining slaves into a more docile, programmable, and controllable group. This mechanism has remained in the human genetic makeup ever since. The engineered gene causes the cervical Atlas (C-1) to dislocate, creating an energy blockage in the spinal column along with a host of physical and mental disturbances.

According to Koven, to this day ninety-nine percent of earth's population is still subject to this ancient curse. The solution is to have the Atlas adjusted back into its perfect position through physical therapy. Chiropractors, doctors, shamans, and practitioners of Atlas Profilax are specially trained to reverse the curse. Ozone injections near the site may also prove to be beneficial.

I have undergone this procedure and can testify to its remarkable healing effects in relieving twenty-five years of pain and stiffness in my neck. Chi kung had helped to loosen and relieve my pain somewhat, but the Atlas Profilax therapy completely corrected and eliminated the pain for a period of three months. One year later I had the procedure done again with the same results. Although the results did not 'hold' for more than three months, the therapy left me with a loose and pain-free neck for a while. I believe the therapy is effective because it releases muscular and tendinous fascial stress, thereby improving blood and lymph oxygenation and allowing sufficient detox of inflammatory substances and complete oxygenation of the injured site. Unfortunately, there are no practitioners of Atlas Profilax within one thousand miles of my home. I am fairly certain that if I was able to have the procedure repeated on a regular basis, my neck would completely and permanently heal.

A dislocated C-1 (Atlas) can certainly affect the continuous free flow of chi into the head, neck, teeth, and jaws, making the Anunnuki curse a viable theory regarding how man has lost the energetic connection with his teeth. Studies show that a misplaced Atlas can disrupt blood flow to the brain stem, setting up an inflammatory process. A misaligned Atlas can also cause a loss of blood circulation to the brain, blood pressure problems, and hinder cerebrospinal fluid circulation and pressure, but it is known that hypertension may be reversed by correcting an Atlas dislocation. A correctly aligned Atlas may well be the KEY to a full recovery to health. The Anunnuki story offers an interesting theory, but the unanswered question still remains:

"Why did humans lose their energetic connection to their teeth?"

In Oriental medicine the kidneys rule the teeth, bones, marrow, and nerves. The role of the kidneys is to store life essence and maintain strong will power. The ability to use our will power to express our unique creativity is dependent on good kidney energy. Strong Kidney Chi gives us the resolve to overcome fear and to pursue our goals. If the kidney energy is weak, our sense of purpose is shaky and we are easily distracted. If the use of teeth, *in any way,* is suppressed or repressed, the Kidney Chi will also be suppressed and repressed. Likewise, if the circular flow of kidney energy to and from the tooth is disrupted in any way, the will power will weaken. And when a tooth is extracted, the kidney energy is depleted and needs to be restored.

Freud suggested that tooth-loss dreams were about—*surprise*—castration. Women also have these dreams, so castration may be gender specific. The general theme in tooth-loss dreams may have to do with a sense of safety, or fear of a loss of self-sufficiency. (In conscious reality, losing a tooth by accident or disease may promote future negative fear-based decision. And such decisions are not in one's best interest and are certainly not in keeping with the way of the warrior.) Castration leads to weakened male energy and castrated males become more docile and less aggressive and have a dampened sense of ambition. Every time I extract a tooth in my dental practice, I have the very uncomfortable feeling that I am castrating the patient. Now you understand one of the reasons why we dentists are so dedicated to saving teeth, why we passionately preach the prevention of tooth and gum disease.

An interesting scientific fact is that teeth 'jiggle' up and down in synchrony with the arterial pulse. Vascular blood pressure within the tooth's arterial network propels the tooth into a positive, outward moving thrust with each heartbeat. There is deep symbolism here: one can suggest that the **teeth connect with will power** and help to drive the positive outward energy of the evolving human consciousness forward. If one's awareness is flowing freely without disruption, one then has the ability to realize one's full potential. Blocking the chi from fully connecting with the teeth, or suppressing and repressing the use of teeth in any way, can be a barrier to self-realization.

In line with this theory, disrupting the flow of chi to the teeth and jaw could suppress a person's will power and ability to freely follow their internal dreams. Someone with insufficient tooth chi will have a difficult time defending themselves from aggressive, controlling dictators. It is easy to see why an overbearing ruler, parent, spouse, or friend could either purposefully or unconsciously endorse artificial taboos on the use of teeth. The 'freedom' of others is dangerous in the eyes of a controlling and power-driven individual.

We can now begin connecting the dots based on science:

— *Teeth are Linked with Kidney Chi and Will Power*
— *A Dislocated Cervical C-1/Atlas Constricts Blood Flow to the Brain Stem, Head, and Teeth*
— *Tooth Loss and/or Limited Capacity due to Constricted Chi Flow is a Symbol for Castration*
— *Docile Personality Combined with Lack of Ambition may be the Result of a Suppressed and/or Repressed Instinct for Defensive Biting*

Docility coupled with a lack of ambition and weakened will power all contribute to the creation of a populace that is easily controlled and afraid to defend itself—qualities despots find desirous in their servants. Psychological and behavioral modification using social taboos renders people more docile and malleable. All the more reason for rulers to create, support and enforce dis-empowering taboos. Man has created many socially driven taboos, and the restrictions on the use of teeth in self-defense stifles the awareness and expression of personal freedoms and inherent rights. A society that unquestioningly accepts the myriad social taboos imposed upon it may find itself at the mercy of a supreme authority willing to subjugate all sense of individual self-determination. We may never discover the true origin of taboos on biting. What is important is awareness of the SOLUTIONS that can free us from the existing universal suppression and repression of this basic instinct.

When we move beyond unproven theories of world domination, we see that teeth hold a sacred responsibility in the evolution of life. Tooth and jaw are certainly critical parts of human anatomy. Tooth, being the hardest substance in the body, is naturally the oldest surviving fossil relic known to man, dating back five hundred million years. I think that there must be a good reason for this amazing resilience. Could it be that nature chose the tooth to hold secrets to man's existence that no other part of the body can preserve? Secrets securely locked and protected by the thick enamel casing of a tooth, secrets about our existence that are yet to be discovered?

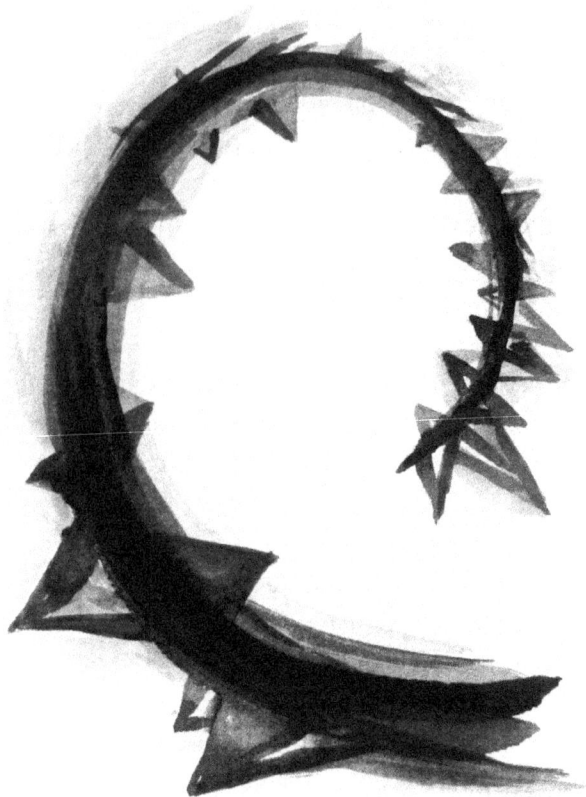

EPILOGUE

During battle to the death in prehistoric days, it is a certainty that these struggles were fought "tooth and nail." Original primal energy was necessarily tapped in order to ensure victory in a vicious fight for life. When a victim is losing the struggle and near death, the last bit of strength remaining will usually go to a futile bite to any exposed and accessible flesh. The mouth is the receptacle for vast amounts of this original primal energy and it is this chi that remains the focus in this book. The sacred mouth sips sweet honey nectar chi, but it can also spit out lethal venomous energy and with its beautiful tongue and teeth can viciously swallow up the life force of another, turning them into slaves, ending their days here on earth.

Man depends on the mouth, teeth, and jaws to feed himself. Early man likely chewed small game such as turtle, frog, snake, fish, bird, and mouse. He did not have the means, at that time, to successfully bring down large game. He certainly could not inflict a lethal bite into the neck of an antelope, wild cat, deer, hog, or other large game animal. Yet his mouth was vital to survival and was packed with large reservoirs of chi, more so than today. That is why I recommend the practice of enhancing the chi of the teeth, tongue, and jaw. One unlocks GREAT potential to increase vital energy and fighting skills by returning to the source.

The first breath of life enters the mouth; mother's milk is taken in at the mouth; the first meal is prepared by chewing with the mouth; the first meaningful sexual encounter usually begins with the mouth. It is the beautiful energy of the mouth that accelerates the breath of life into our dreams and the life and dreams of our brothers and sisters. And so neglect and misuse of the mouth necessarily engenders weakness and disease.

There is a spiritual power to the teeth, tongue, and jaw that is both respected and feared by those who know it. Many cultures from the past held deer teeth in high regard and buried their dead with them, and to date archaeologists have uncovered graves fifteen thousand years old containing hundreds of red deer canine teeth. Deer teeth are spiritual relics that symbolized hunting and one's ability to provide for others. It makes good sense, in today's world, to focus and meditate on our own teeth in the hope that we may perhaps reveal the valuable secrets we subconsciously hold. The understanding of spirit, in my opinion, is critical to all martial artists. We need to connect with it, understand it, and be able to draw from it when necessary.

I sincerely hope that this book stimulates you to further investigate the role that the teeth and jaws play in our ultimate survival and in the fulfillment of our individual destinies. It is our duty to break the shackles imposed by 'polite society'—which, in my opinion, are no less than a type of enforced castration—and make peace with this most basic of instincts that is necessary for our imminent survival. Martial artists who take the time to cultivate the chi of the teeth and jaws will simultaneously improve their fighting skills and overall health. And most importantly, we clear the path to our own self-realization and possibly grant ourselves the freedom to save our lives or the lives of those we love.